ABOUT THE AUTHOR

Maryon Stewart studied preventive dentistry and nutrition at the Royal Dental Hospital in London and worked as a counsellor with nutritional doctors in England for four years. At the beginning of 1984 she set up the PMT Advisory Service which has subsequently helped thousands of women world-wide. In 1987 she launched the Women's Nutritional Advisory Service which now provides broader help to women of all ages.

Maryon Stewart is the author of the best-selling books *No More PMS!*, now in its Third Edition, *Beat Sugar Craving*, *Beat the Menopause Without HRT*, *Healthy Parents, Healthy Baby*, *The Natural Health Bible* and *Maryon Stewart's Zest for Life Plan*. She is the co-author of *No More IBS!* and *The PMS Cookbook* and. She has had her own weekly radio programme on health and nutrition; she has co-written several medical papers, and has written articles for many glossy magazines, including *Marie Claire*, *Cosmopolitan*, *Chat*, *Woman's Journal*, *BBC Good Health*, *Woman's Own*, *Health & Fitness* and for both *The Daily Mirror* and *Daily Mail*.

She has also appeared on several popular TV magazine shows, such as TV AM, GMTV, Top of the Morning, Channel Four Food File, BBC Here & Now, Good Morning with Anne & Nick, Reportage, Meridian, Carlton, MSkyB, The Miriam Stoppard Health & Beauty Show, This Morning, Pebble Mill, Channel Four, Streetwise and TVS. She has contributed regularly to Capital Woman, has done a series of pro- grammes for Yorkshire TVs Help Yourself programmes and has helped Anglia TV with their Bodyworks series. Maryon has written her own regular page in the magazines *House and Garden*, *Healthy Eating and Good Health*, and now writes regular articles for both the national daily newspapers and women's magazines. She is also on the Expert Panel of Contributors for *Top Santé* magazine and frequently lectures to both the lay public and medical profession. In a *Good Housekeeping* survey pub- lished in November 1999, she was voted the 51st most influential woman in Great Britain. She is married to Dr Alan Stewart; they live in Lewes, Sussex, with their four children.

D0318593

CRUISING THROUGH THE **MENOPAUSE**

*Managing your menopause
successfully without HRT*

Maryon Stewart

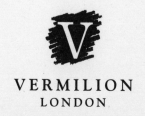

VERMILION
LONDON

To my mother, Rosa, with eternal love

First published in Great Britain in 2000

1 3 5 7 9 10 8 6 4 2

Text copyright © Maryon Stewart 1995, 1997, 2000

Maryon Stewart has asserted her right to be identified as the author of
this work under the Copyright, Designs and Patents Act 1988.

All rights reserved. No part of this publication may be reproduced,
stored in a retrieval system, or transmitted in any form or by any means,
electronic, mechanical, photocopying, recording or otherwise, without
the prior permission of the copyright owner.

First published in 1995 as *Beat the Menopause without HRT* by Headline
Book Publishing
A second edition published in 1997 by Headline Book Publishing

This updated edition published in 2000 by Vermilion,
an imprint of Ebury Press
Random House
20 Vauxhall Bridge Road
London SW1V 2SA

Random House South Africa (Pty) Limited
Endulini, 5A Jubilee Road,
Parktown 2193, South Africa

The Random House Group Limited Reg. No. 954009

www.randomhouse.co.uk

A CIP catalogue record for this book is available from the
British Library

ISBN: 0 09 185650 7

Papers used by Vermilion are natural, recyclable products made from
wood grown in sustainable forests.

Printed and bound by Biddles of Guildford

CONTENTS

May you live all the days of your life

Jonathan Swift (1667–1745)

IMPORTANT NOTE

Many fairly technical terms are used to describe the phases of the menopause and its associated conditions. While many of the terms are explained in the text, you will find a Dictionary of Terms on page 311. It is important to have a good understanding of the text, so do look words up, even if you are only vaguely unsure of their meaning.

Also, although every effort has been made to ensure that the contents of this book are accurate, it must not be treated as a substitute for qualified medical advice. Always consult a qualified medical practitioner. Neither the Author nor the Publisher can be held responsible for any loss or claim arising out of the use, or misuse, of the suggestions made or the failure to take medical advice.

ACKNOWLEDGEMENTS

Were it not for published research from around the world, the Women's Nutritional Advisory Service (WNAS) programme for the menopause would probably never have come about. So, my first round of gratitude must go to the many academics who have collectively pioneered the non-drug approach to alleviating the symptoms of the menopause, and preserving long-term health. Although the list is too long to mention them all, many of their names are listed in the reference section which begins on page 328. However, I cannot move on without thanking Drs Lorraine Dennerstein, Alice Murkies and Wilcox from Australia, Professor Kenneth Setchell and Drs Guy Abraham and Notelovitz from the USA, Professor Hermann Adlercreutz from Finland, plus Drs Whitehead and Myra Hunter from the UK – their collective work has been invaluable.

Special thanks must go to Dr Alan Stewart, my partner in all senses of the word, for his valuable technical support, without which we would not have been able to provide such valuable help to so many women, or education on the scientifically based non-drug approach to so many health-care professionals.

Sincere thanks must go next to the wonderful patients who have volunteered to share their personal stories with us in this book, in a quest to help others suffering similarly. Their willingness to relate their past experiences, no matter how painful, even before they knew I intended to change their names, is hugely appreciated.

A million thanks go to my team at the WNAS who have jointly helped to make this book possible. Helen Heap, our nutritionist, for contributing greatly to the recipe section, and helping to document the personal stories and the appendices, among other last-minute activities. Gillian Byrne, our nurse, for conducting her share of the consultations that resulted in 'case histories'. Cheryl Griffiths for keeping my plate from running over; Julie Anne McWhinne for her help with the latest GP survey and updates on new research while visiting from Australia; and to Lisa Graham for taking pride in manning the WNAS helpline.

I am also exceedingly grateful to Laura Topper MSc for writing such a down-to-earth chapter on the benefits of exercise, and for the advice I received from Deryn Bell on osteopathy, from Paul Lundberg on acupuncture, and from Julia Barker on herbal medicine.

A tip of the hat also goes to Charlotte Howard, my literary agent, for her professionalism and sense of humour and to Joanna Carreras from Vermilion, for both her vision and expert editing.

Liz Copping and Jackie Hartt need oodles of acknowledgement for their help with the children and the household chores while I was engrossed in the book. The children themselves: Phoebe, Chesney, Hester and Simeon, need a loud cheer for allowing me the time to get the words on the page, and for providing everything from words of encouragement to back rubs and hugs.

And lastly, how do I thank Alan, my dear husband, who lovingly prepared the sustenance to keep me going while I was writing, wrote the chapter on Hormone Replacement Therapy and remained supportive until the final draft was printed. You can be sure he will be rewarded with ongoing love and gratitude.

I may take the bow, but it was a true team effort!

Maryon Stewart
May 2000

FOREWORD

The menopause is something which must come to every woman, and this 'change of life' unfortunately brings with it a number of problems. The readjustments that take place within the body at this time can cause hot flushes, sleeplessness and irritability amongst many symptoms, and can lead the way to other conditions, not least osteoporosis, the fragile bone disease to which so many women over fifty fall victim.

Up until very recently it seemed as though the medical establishment was blind to the problems of women of that certain age, and our mothers and grandmothers would have had to suffer in silence. With the advent of hormone replacement therapy (HRT), however, everything appeared to be solved, and women felt they could look forward to a middle and old age free of all the symptoms they anticipated with dread. At last the spectre of the menopause had been banished from their futures.

But had it? Well, no, for some women the spectre remained. Just as every woman has a different reaction to the hormonal upheavals that take place in the body during the menopause, so women had different reactions to the various constituents of the pills or patches of HRT. Some experienced symptoms even worse than those of the menopause they were trying to evade; many others disliked the idea of chemical interference anyway; but even more women were actually unable to take HRT, for a variety of health reasons, some quite serious – in my case the risk associated with breast cancer.

It was then that the cavalry arrived, in the shape of the Women's Nutritional Advisory Service and in the person of Maryon Stewart. Having spent a dozen or so years studying the effects of the pre-menstrual syndrome (PMS) on women, she knew that a natural rather than a chemical approach was the answer, and realized that the same principles could be applied to the problems involved in the menopause. It could be faced through means other than HRT.

Her emphasis on weight-bearing exercise and a more active lifestyle, plenty of relaxation, sensible nutritional supplementation and on eating good natural foods makes for a healthy framework for living that could last well beyond the years of the menopause. *Cruising Through the Menopause* is a book that every woman should buy, read and follow. The rest of their lives could depend on it.

Diana Moran
London, 2000

INTRODUCTION
THE WNAS EXPERIENCE

Women can overcome the symptoms of the menopause without having to resort to taking Hormone Replacement Therapy. Sixteen years of helping women over their health problems at the Women's Nutritional Advisory Service (WNAS) allows me to put my hand on my heart and state with certainty that there is an effective scientifically based natural alternative. Published research now clearly supports the fact that menopausal symptoms can be overcome without having to resort to HRT, and at the same time protect us from both heart disease and the bone-thinning disease osteoporosis in the longer term. Despite this, the alternative approach is not widely known about outside medical research circles, and is certainly not widely practised by doctors, largely through ignorance.

Over the last 14 years, we at the WNAS have pioneered an exceedingly simple, workable and enjoyable programme to help to alleviate the symptoms of both the perimenopause and the menopause, no matter how severe. The success rate, within a matter of months, astounds most of the patients, and is a constant source of satisfaction to our team of health professionals. Although I get enormous satisfaction from helping individuals over their symptoms, the success brings with it a great deal of frustration. Knowing that there is a workable alternative, based on sound research and extensive clinical practice, I constantly despair about the millions of women around the world who are left on what I call 'the medical scrap heap', to fend for themselves, not realising that there are simple and effective measures that they can implement which will alleviate their symptoms within a matter of weeks or months.

The purpose of *Cruising Through the Menopause* is to explain clearly about the pros and cons of taking HRT, including when and if it should be taken, and to spread the word about the workability of the WNAS programme to women everywhere, enabling them to make informed choices and thus remain in the driving seat throughout their menopause. I am sure you will agree that it is highly desirable to remain

11

in good health for what may turn out to be the second half of your life. These days women are living so much longer, on average reaching their mid-eighties and in many cases far beyond. It is therefore vitally important that we become familiar with all the self-help measures that science provides, not just to overcome the distressing menopausal symptoms but additionally to preserve the health of our heart, our bones and our mental well-being in the long-term.

To this day, Hormone Replacement Therapy remains the treatment of choice for most doctors for both perimenopausal and menopausal women. This is mainly because, by their own admission, they were under-educated on the subject of nutrition as undergraduates, and most of their post-graduate education has come from the pharmaceutical companies, many of whom are the HRT producers. This may be fine for the women who feel happy and well taking HRT. However, research shows that up to two-thirds of women who try HRT come off it within the first year because of side-effects or dissatisfaction. In addition, there are women who cannot take HRT for a variety of medical reasons, as you will see from Chapter 5 and, indeed, for some women HRT is not an option they would willingly consider. Despite this, according to the results of our recent survey of a thousand GPs (see page 75), very few doctors are equipped with the knowledge to provide scientifically based alternative advice. So even now, despite the wealth of published papers on the non-drug approach to the menopause, many women are either locked in to taking HRT whether they like it or not, or left to fend for themselves.

Repeated WNAS surveys on menopausal women constantly confirm the fear and confusion women experience about the changes and symptoms that accompany the menopause, and the prospect of becoming a victim of the bone-thinning disease, osteoporosis. These days we often encounter conflicting reports about the pros and cons of HRT and the workability of alternative approaches, both in scientific journals and the media. *Cruising Through the Menopause* is designed to put an end to the confusion by presenting the scientific evidence in easily understandable terms. For, once you have the facts at your fingertips, you will be armed with all the information you need in order to make the choices with which you feel happy.

A SNAPSHOT OF THE WNAS PROGRAMME

Over the last 14 years, we have helped thousands of women through their perimenopause and helped even more to overcome their menopausal symptoms. Our programme has become increasingly successful as science has provided us with even more workable tools. In Part 4 of *Cruising Through the Menopause*, I have presented the 'secrets' behind the WNAS programme, so that you can devise a programme to help you through your perimenopause and indeed to overcome your menopausal symptoms. As you work your way through the book you will discover that the WNAS programme we have devised over the years consists mainly of the following:

1 Making specific dietary changes including:
   • improving the nutrient content of the diet and removing foods that may impede the absorption of good nutrients
   • removing from the diet those foods that will worsen the hot flushes and night sweats
   • including in the diet those foods that are rich in phytoestrogens (naturally occuring oestrogens), which are Mother Nature's way of allowing us to top up on natural oestrogen on a daily basis.
2 Taking nutritional supplements including vitamins, minerals, herbs and a phytoestrogen-rich supplement, which have proved their worth in clinical trials
3 Doing moderate weight-bearing exercise to stimulate the brain chemistry and to help keep both heart and bones in a healthy condition
4 Following a regular relaxation programme which dramatically reduces hot flushes and helps to keep you feeling in control.

In addition, there are numerous menu plans, both for meat eaters and vegetarians, and more than 80 delicious recipes to incorporate into your repertoire if you enjoy cooking. If you are not one of life's devoted cooks, or have little time to spend in the kitchen, then you will enjoy numerous fast, but nutritious, options, which take very little time to prepare, but will still provide you with the needed nutrients.

WHY DO WOMEN SUFFER AT THE MENOPAUSE?

In order to understand what happens in the body at the time of the menopause, it is first necessary to go back in time to the child-bearing years. Many physical demands are placed upon us in these years, which can result in poor health prospects when not met. At the WNAS, we know from our own research on women of child-bearing age with premenstrual syndrome (PMS), that between 50 and 80 per cent of them have a shortage of an important mineral called magnesium, and other nutrients such as B vitamins, iron, zinc and essential fatty acids.

Let's use magnesium as an example. It's needed for:

- Normal brain chemical metabolism (and brain chemistry can be likened to the conductor of an orchestra – it is he/she who ultimately determines harmony)
- Normal hormone function
- Smooth muscle control (both the uterus and the gut are smooth muscles)

It stands to reason, therefore, that a shortage of magnesium alone can influence both physical and mental well-being, all aspects of our menstrual cycle, and our gut function.

Extra nutrient demands are also placed on women's bodies during pregnancy, and even more so when breast-feeding. Mother Nature in her wisdom ensures that the growing baby gets all the nutrients needed for development, which means they go sailing across the placenta and through the breast milk, often leaving the mother in a poor nutritional state.

As years go by, levels of some nutrients in women's bodies naturally reduce. By the time we reach the menopause we are often in a nutritionally depleted state, effectively firing on two cylinders instead of four. As the menopause is such a major transition in a woman's life, the body needs to be in good shape in order to ensure a smooth passage, and because of these nutritional imbalances, many women can experience uncomfortable and disturbing symptoms. For instance, the hot flushes that are experienced at the time of the menopause are simply the result of brain chemistry attempting to kick-start the ovaries back into function. When our natural oestrogen levels have fallen as a result of dwindling ovarian function, consuming foods that contain naturally occurring oestrogen, and improving nutritional status through diet and lifestyle, influences brain chemistry positively, and as a result hot flushes and nightsweats dramatically subside.

Later in the book you'll read about the survey we conducted on 500 women who had recently been through the menopause. We found their symptoms broke down into three separate categories. The first group, perhaps the most obvious, had the oestrogen-withdrawal symptoms: hot flushes, nightsweats, dry vagina and insomnia. These symptoms were directly related to falling oestrogen levels in the body.

We call the remaining two groups 'physical symptoms' – aches, pains, migraines, palpitations, headaches, irritable bowel syndrome and fatigue – and 'mental symptoms' – panic attacks, mood swings, aggression and depression. Most interestingly, the survey revealed that both the 'physical' and the 'mental' symptoms were more related to dietary and lifestyle inadequacies than they were to falling oestrogen levels in the body. Another survey conducted on 200 menopause patients in 1997 echoed this: it showed that physical and mental symptoms were more commonly suffered at the time of the menopause than oestrogen withdrawal symptoms.

This was an extraordinary finding, and one which lies at the heart of our advice about the menopause and its treatment. Now that we can appreciate the symptoms experienced at the menopause are not necessarily all to do with falling oestrogen levels, perhaps our expectations of HRT, as a result of its media image, are too high. HRT is designed mainly to counteract the oestrogen-withdrawal symptoms rather than the 'physical' and 'mental' symptoms we have now identified. The WNAS programme aims to address *all* these groups of symptoms effectively. One audit on patients who have been through our programme, showed that 85 per cent of women feel that their menopause symptoms are under control within four months (Group 1, oestrogen-withdrawal symptoms) and 90 per cent report having overcome 'physical' and 'mental' symptoms within the same time period. Results of other audits are detailed throughout the book.

When we redress the balance and put back in the body what time and nature have taken out, it seems to have a normalising effect on brain chemistry and hormone function. It is a bit like turning the factory lights back on. It is almost as if the women return to their pre-menopausal condition.

Having treated thousands of patients over the years at the WNAS, I have witnessed many wonderful transformations as women regain their quality of health, confidence and self-esteem. Our 'case histories', who have generously shared their stories with us in this book, are a few typical examples.

« Molly's Story »

Molly was a forty-nine-year-old mother of two from Potters Bar in Hertfordshire. When she approached the WNAS for help she was taking prescribed hormones and was experiencing severe PMS symptoms as a side-effect.

'As my periods diminished the hot flushes began. By the time my periods stopped altogether I was experiencing horrendous night sweats, at least two or three times a night, with never a night off. I also suffered tingling and numbness in my arms and legs, loss of confidence, vitality and ability to concentrate. I became aggressive, had water retention, breast tenderness, fatigue, aching legs, was hypersensitive to music and light, had alternating bouts of constipation and diarrhoea, plus flatulence, migraine, depression and itchy skin that had bothered me for years.

My doctor prescribed Prempack-C which seemed OK at first but after approximately three months I was experiencing headaches and progressively heavier bleeding, so much so that even two night-time sanitary towels together would not cope.

After six months my doctor changed my hormone preparation to Syntex Menophase, which again was fine at the start. After a few months I began experiencing cramps for two days and nights each month, and severe PMS, worse than anything I had ever known before. I felt so wretched before my monthly bleed that I did not want to go out or see anyone. For this reason my doctor then prescribed progesterone pessaries. I used one each morning for three days, but these made me feel as if I was enveloped in a net shroud so that I felt completely detached from what was happening around me. I also gained about ten pounds while on the HRT.

My attitude to my family changed. I became very grudging, not wanting to do anything for anyone. A resentful attitude pervaded everything I did. I was very bad-tempered with my husband and generally unhappy. I often wrote myself notes to remind me of things to nag him about when he came home from work.

I reached rock bottom one evening when I was tired and hungry while cooking dinner. My husband insisted on questioning me despite my telling him to leave me alone until after I had eaten. He persisted, saying he needed an immediate answer. I picked up a sharp pointed kitchen knife and thrust it at his abdomen. Fortunately for both of us it was winter and the knife did not seriously penetrate his layers of clothing.

I was relieved to learn about the work of the WNAS while watching a lunchtime television programme and subsequently enrolled on their postal and telephone services. Initially I bought the book No More PMS! And began to follow its recommendations. Once I had completed the questionnaire and diet diary sent to me by the WNAS, they wrote a programme for me which I immediately began to follow. I reduced my intake of wheat, sugar, salt, tea, coffee, alcohol, chocolate and spicy food. On the third day withdrawal symptoms started, mainly headaches, and lasted for four days. After this my symptoms began lifting and I knew I was heading in the right direction. I also took the supplements Gynovite Plus and vitamin E, and followed a moderate *weight-bearing exercise programme. That was four years ago. Now I am more stable and things do not bug me like they used to. Within three months of starting the programme, I was told that I was a much nicer person than I had been for years. I really think that if I had not followed the WNAS programme, I would now be in Holloway Prison serving a sentence for murder!'*

Molly and the many other case histories who have kindly agreed to appear in this book will reassure you that you are not suffering alone and will give you hope that the end of your symptoms is in sight. Realistically, you need to devote the next four to six months to helping yourself back into good health. According to our research, the extent to which you follow the recommendations is directly related to your recovery rate. Once you have read through the book and worked out the programme to follow, stick to it like superglue!

If you feel you can't manage alone and would like some extra help or advice, then you will find the address of the WNAS on page 309. It's never too early to improve your general health and to work towards preventing osteoporosis. So, as you approach menopausal age, even if you are symptom-free, work out a diet that you would find enjoyable, using the guidelines given later in the book, together with a moderate exercise and nutritional supplement regime. If you start in time you might even sail through the menopause without noticing it!

Whether you are approaching the perimenopause, currently in the throes of the menopause, or have just emerged from it, you will need to read the first parts of the book and then go on to work out your tailor-made programme from the guidelines in Parts Three and Four. You will also find daily menus and delicious recipes to try there, as well as notes on the nutritional content of food: this will help you to choose the foods you like, knowing that they are rich in the essential vitamins and minerals.

Finding the programme that your body thrives on is a voyage of discovery that need only be made once. It's a voyage that both you and your family will undoubtedly be glad you undertook as you once again experience good health and well-being.

Good luck and *bon voyage*.

Menopause Symptom Questionnaire

Do you suffer from any of the following? Please ensure each symptom is only ticked once.

MOLLY	* How many times per month	None	Mild	Moderate	Severe
1 Hot/cold flushes*	Too many to count				✓
2 Facial/body flushing*					✓
3 Nightsweats*					✓
4 Palpitations*			✓		
5 Panic attacks*			✓		
6 Generalised aches and pains				✓	
7 Depression			✓		
8 Perspiration			✓		
9 Numbness/skin tingling in arms and legs		✓			
10 Headaches				✓	
11 Backaches				✓	
12 Fatigue				✓	
13 Irritability				✓	
14 Anxiety				✓	
15 Nervousness				✓	
16 Loss of confidence					✓
17 Insomnia					
18 Giddiness/dizziness		✓			
19 Difficulty/frequency in passing water				✓	
20 Water retention					✓

21	Bloated abdomen			
22	Constipation		✓	
23	Itchy vagina			✓
24	Dry vagina			✓
25	Painful intercourse			
26	Decreased sex drive			
27	Loss of concentration	✓		
28	Confusion/Loss of vitality	✓		

Have you noticed since the onset of the menopause:

1 Loss of height   Yes ☑ No ☐

2 Difficulty in bending   Yes ☑ No ☐

3 Increased curvature of back   Yes ☑ No ☐

Are any of the above symptoms cyclic? (i.e. come in cycles, for example on a monthly basis   I have not noticed

Have you gained weight since you started the menopause?   Yes ☑ No ☐   If yes, how much   7–10 lb

Do you have any other menopausal symptoms not mentioned above? _____

How long have you had menopausal symptoms?   18 months

Did you suffer from pre-menstrual tension prior to the menopause?   Yes ☑ No ☐   If yes, for how long? _____

Follow-up Menopause Questionnaire

Do you suffer from any of the following? Please ensure each symptom is only ticked *once*.

MOLLY	* How many times per month	None	Mild	Moderate	Severe
1 Hot/cold flushes*	1–3 per day		✓		
2 Facial/body flushing*			✓		
3 Nightsweats*		✓			
4 Palpitations*		✓			
5 Panic attacks*		✓			
6 Generalised aches and pains		✓			
7 Depression		✓			
8 Perspiration		✓			
9 Numbness/skin tingling in arms and legs		✓			
10 Headaches		✓			
11 Backaches		✓			
12 Fatigue			✓		
13 Irritability			✓		
14 Anxiety		✓			
15 Nervousness		✓			
16 Loss of confidence		✓			
17 Insomnia		✓			
18 Giddiness/dizziness		✓			
19 Difficulty/frequency in passing water		✓			
20 Water retention		✓			

21	Bloated abdomen	✓	
22	Constipation	✓	
23	Itchy vagina	✓	
24	Dry vagina	✓	
25	Painful intercourse		
26	Decreased sex drive		
27	Loss of concentration		✓
28	Confusion/Loss of vitality	✓	

Are any of the above symptoms cyclic? (i.e. come in cycles, for example on a monthly basis) *I don't know, none are bad enough to be a problem*

PART ONE

MENOPAUSE – THE LONG AND THE SHORT OF IT

1

THE PERIMENOPAUSE BEGINS ITS VOYAGE

At the time of the menopause the leisure and pleasure years should stretch joyously before you. Now that women are living longer than ever before, there are golden opportunities to indulge in all the leisure pursuits that may have taken your fancy and achieve some of the goals that were just dreams when family and work commitments took a priority. When the family are old enough to be independent and the financial commitments have dwindled, in theory there should be no stopping you so long as you are in good health.

However, for at least three-quarters of all women, the menopause brings with it rapid changes and unwanted symptoms which, in many cases, are life-disrupting and produce utter misery. Being reduced to a hot, red, anxious, introverted wreck, struggling to keep a grip on life at the very time when it should be at its peak, is a bitter pill to swallow.

Until recently the menopause has been shrouded in secrecy, a near taboo subject that was hardly discussed in public. Who wants to admit that they are 'at the beginning of the end' and having a rough time? As we live longer, it stands to reason that we shall survive experiences that perhaps previous generations did not encounter. How should we cope with this? Who should we turn to for answers, when the medical profession are perhaps not fully equipped to deal with them? The menopause can be and has been for many women both a frightening and an isolating experience.

In a sense, we are pioneers, and there are lots of thus-far unanswered questions which I shall address in this book. Here you will find the myths of menopause uncovered and the pros and cons of HRT unveiled. You will learn about the hormonal changes that occur at the time of the menopause and why they rob you of your confidence, your 'cool' and your libido. After reading Parts One and Two you will be able to stand back and make some informed choices for yourself, feeling secure about your new knowledge and the fact that you are in control of your body.

For those who can or wish to take Hormone Replacement Therapy (HRT), a rapid solution may be in sight. However, for those who cannot tolerate HRT, either for medical reasons or because of the many side-effects, or for those who do not wish to take it, the medical profession has little to offer to allay symptoms and to help prevent the silent bone-thinning disease, osteoporosis.

All in all, I estimate that for up to 50 per cent of women, HRT is not an option in the long term. A large proportion of women do not take hormones as a solution to their menopausal symptoms. Estimates of usage in countries such as Italy, France, Germany, Denmark, South Australia, the UK and the USA, range from three per cent in Italy to 32 per cent in California. Many women who begin using hormone therapy abandon it within a few months: according to one study the average duration of therapy is nine months and of those who start treatment, up to two-thirds will abandon it within one year. It therefore follows that there has to be a scientifically based alternative.

YOU AND THE MENOPAUSE

The word menopause does not mean it's the beginning of the end or a pause between men! Simply translated, it actually means the end of the monthly fertility cycle. The term was coined by a French physician called Gardanne, who referred to it in 1812 as *menepausie* and subsequently shortened it to *menopause* in 1821. The word menopause comes from the Greek *meno*, meaning 'month', and *pausis*, which means 'ending' or, more literally, 'a pause in a life-cycle'.

Throughout the years, this 'pause' has been vilified, misunderstood, dreaded . . . But now, fortunately for all of us, we have a much better understanding of the workings of the body, and the ways in which we can influence our brain chemicals and hormones by improving our nutritional state. Although hormone replacement is still a favourite first-line therapy in some quarters, there are now other proven approaches to overcoming menopausal symptoms and preventing osteoporosis. As modern women, who have an equal voice in society, we now have a choice.

WHAT YOUR MOTHER DIDN'T TELL YOU

We were taught about contraception at school and given information about having children. During pregnancy we were bombarded with information and choices about where and how to have our babies. Our mothers and their friends gave advice at every available opportunity, hoping to pass on their wisdom and make life easier for us. So why is it that we are all in the dark about the menopause? The menopause is a natural event, after all, not a disease, and it affects one-half of the world's population!

In the UK alone more than 13 million women are over 40 and it's estimated that this will increase by a further one and a half million by the year 2001. In the USA statistics show that between 40 and 50 million women will pass through the 'change of life' by the year 2000. Here in the UK and also in Australia, according to Theresa Gorman MP, one-third of the hospital beds are occupied by women who have a menopausal-related problem. That must signify that the menopause and osteoporosis, the bone-thinning disease that affects one out of every three women, are causing serious problems which are not being sufficiently addressed in preventive terms.

Many of our mothers' generation would not have been brought up on free communication. Before the 1960s, most women only spoke about their most personal and intimate problems behind closed doors. The average Victorian woman's expectation was to keep reproducing almost until she died. The average age expectancy was approximately 55 years, so there was therefore little need for society to make preparations to see women through the menopause and beyond.

Now that we live far longer than previous generations – the average lifespan for a woman is currently 83 – it means that at the time of the menopause we still have on average 40 per cent of our lives left to live. This completely scotches the myth that by the start of the menopause we are already in God's waiting-room!

On the whole, women do not sit at home any more producing large families and waiting on their nearest and dearest. They have careers, pursue hobbies and are expected to remain productive members of society well into their sixties and even their seventies. Women of 50 in the 1990s simply don't look like women of a similar age 50 years ago. We not only look younger, we feel younger, which may be why the menopause often takes us by surprise. I've often heard women say 'I'm not old enough to be menopausal', but that is largely due to their preconceived ideas. In a recent survey we conducted on menopausal women, the youngest to start her menopause was only 23 years old! Admittedly that is abnormally young because the average age is 50, but it can happen at any time. We just have to prepare ourselves mentally and make sure that we are in the best possible shape.

Our expectations and perception of ourselves have also changed dramatically. These days, women in their forties and fifties are not on the social scrap-heap. It is quite acceptable for women of menopausal age to keep up with fashion trends if they so desire and to actively work to maintain their youthful appearance. There is even the extreme option of having faces lifted, breasts enlarged, and other little discreet tucks, purses permitting, all of which are procedures that didn't even occur in the wildest dreams of past generations. In the 1990s, thanks to Emmeline Pankhurst and her colleagues, women sit in boardrooms, they stand for parliament, they perform operations, they climb mountains and compete with men on a day-to-day basis. They do not expect to retire into the woodwork from the time of their first hot flush or expect to take a two-year sabbatical to have their menopause in peace.

Thankfully, medical science has moved on tremendously in the lifetime of our generation. We are far more enlightened about the causes of potentially fatal conditions like heart disease, cancer and indeed osteoporosis, and we are beginning to understand how we can prevent these diseases from taking over and bringing an abrupt end to our lives.

It is all a question of perception. Your expectations of your menopause may well influence the kind of menopause you experience. With this in mind, in 1994 we conducted a survey of 500 women who had recently experienced their menopause, to examine their attitudes, hopes and fears about the menopause as it approached.

SURVEY RESULTS

- 80 per cent of women reported that they were delighted that their periods had stopped. This was by far the most agreed-upon factor.
- 45 per cent looked forward to more leisure time.
- 40 per cent said they were afraid that their physical appearance would disintegrate quickly.
- 37 per cent felt that the menopause signalled the start of old age!
- 33 per cent thought it was right 'to grow old gracefully'.
- 19 per cent were willing to trade youth for wisdom.
- 35 per cent were pleased they no longer needed to use contraception.
- 32 per cent felt positive about the start of a new era.
- 28 per cent felt pleased that they could look forward to pursuing their own goals.
- 17 per cent dreaded their menopause.
- 8 per cent found it difficult to come to terms with no longer being fertile.

- 17 per cent wondered if their partner would now prefer a younger woman.
- 14 per cent felt sexually liberated.

THE WOMAN'S REALM SURVEY

For many years the Women's Nutritional Advisory Service have been approached by women for advice about diet and lifestyle around the time of the menopause. In the early 1980s we felt that we did not really have enough information to give much solid and useful advice to many of these women.

Gradually our opinion has changed, and for several good reasons. First, the value of hormone replacement therapy has become much better defined. Its benefits and risks are now quite well understood although there remain some important unanswered questions, and we know also what it is good for and what it is not so good for. It is clear that for some women it is not the answer and in the UK in particular there is a degree of reluctance to use HRT by both doctors and the public.

Second, the last 10 years have seen the publication of many scientific papers documenting the relationship between nutrition and hormone function. Could this explain the enormous variation in hormone levels within the normal female population and the great individual variation in response to some hormone treatments for menopausal-related and other symptoms?

Finally, our own experience and that of others in treating women with premenstrual syndrome led us to conclude that diet and lifestyle had a major impact on both the physical and mental symptoms of these women. Some of them began to come back saying, 'You helped me with my PMS. Now that I am approaching the menopause, what can I do to help control my own symptoms?' Gradually, from listening to these women, understanding their symptoms and advising them along lines similar to those that had helped them with their premenstrual problems, we were able to see that dietary and lifestyle factors could also be important in the menopause.

We wanted to know more. Over the years tens of thousands of women have contacted us about PMS, but because of our caution our contact with women around the time of the menopause was rather limited. We knew, like most research scientists, that if you really want to know what is going on, you will have to collect information from hundreds of women. The reason for this is that around the time of the menopause there are many factors to be considered. These include age at the time of the menopause (strictly speaking the date of the last natural period), gynaecological history, especially if there has been a hysterectomy, dietary factors, the influence of stress, the role that their partner might play, and so on.

We were very pleased when Gill Cox at *Woman's Realm* agreed to help us by publishing a questionnaire for women at the time of the menopause. Kimberly-Clark helped with funding to analyse the results of the survey and kindly offered all the respondents a sample of their panty-liners. Efamol also kindly financially supported our research into the menopause.

We have been enormously helped by this survey which has brought forward our understanding of menopausal symptoms and their relationship to dietary and lifestyle factors. The results are to be found in the relevant chapters throughout this book and especially in the following three.

The response to the survey was excellent. After it appeared in a February issue we soon had the 500 replies we had hoped for and set about analysing the findings. Each woman was asked more than 30 questions, many with several subsections, so that in all we had nearly a hundred pieces of information from each woman.

Of the first 500 replies, only 418 revealed their age! Who did they think we were going to tell? Their average age at the time of their last period was 46 years; the youngest was 23 and the oldest 57. This sample had experienced their menopause some four years earlier than the general population.

Age at the time of the menopause

Age in years	23–30	31–40	41–45	46–50	51–55	56+
% of women in survey	1	16	27	40	15	1

Time since their last period

Time since last period	Under 4	4–6	7–12	13–24	25–48	49–72	73–120	121–372
% of women	22	5	6	15	14	12	13	13

The average time since the last period was four years and eight months or fifty-six months.

Changes in periods

40.4 per cent commented that their periods became irregular as they approached the menopause. Furthermore, 44 per cent marked the questionnaire to say that their periods had become heavier, 17 per cent to say that they had become lighter, and 39 per cent that there had been no change with this aspect of their periods.

Hysterectomy

Of the 500 women, 119 (23.8 per cent) had previously had a hysterectomy, but oddly enough, over one-third were not sure whether their ovaries were intact or not! You can bet their bodies knew.

Relationship between age and symptoms

Although we looked at 12 different symptoms, only hot flushes showed any relationship. The younger that women were at the time of the menopause, the more likely they were to be troubled by hot flushes. It would thus seem that the younger you are at the time of the change, the less easily it is tolerated. But this is not quite true, as hot flushes were the only symptom to show this pattern; no other symptom was influenced by age. This was our first clear indication that there was something more than just a change in hormones involved. This is a view increasingly supported by other researchers.

2

SET SAIL FOR THE MENOPAUSE

THE NORMAL MENSTRUAL CYCLE

Approximately each month under normal circumstances, our ovaries produce an egg ready for fertilisation. This happens under the stimulus and direction of hormones produced by the pituitary gland which is situated at the base of the brain, a few inches behind our eyes. It produces many hormones to control the thyroid gland in the neck, and the adrenal glands in the abdomen and the ovaries. It has been likened to the conductor of a hormonal orchestra. It controls hormone output by these glands on a day-to-day and even minute-to-minute basis. The ovary, for its part, provides two main elements; the eggs which come pre-formed as Graafian follicles (named after their discoverer), and the *theca* or substance of the ovary in which the tiny follicles are embedded and which is responsible for the production of the female sex hormones, oestrogen and progesterone.

The ovary has a limited supply of eggs, all of which were formed in the womb before your own birth – hence the importance of your mother's health and diet during pregnancy. Each month, several follicles are stimulated to develop by a hormone from the pituitary appropriately called follicle-stimulating hormone (FSH). Usually one follicle, matures to a point where an egg is released, an event that normally takes place in the middle of the cycle. The egg is released as a result of a small rise in FSH, and a very large surge of a second hormone from the pituitary called luteinising hormone (LH).

In the first part of the cycle, the ovaries are also busy producing oestrogen which encourages the lining of the womb to thicken so that it might be ready should fertilisation take place. Oestrogen levels continue at a moderate level after ovulation and are joined by the second female sex hormone, progesterone. This is produced by the follicle in the ovary after the egg has been released and reaches a substantial peak around day 21 of the cycle. It then falls away unless fertilisation takes place, and the rapid fall in the level of progesterone causes the lining of the womb to be shed and a period results.

So these two key hormones from the pituitary, FSH and LH, dictate the events in the ovary in terms of whether ovulation will take place or not and how much of the hormones oestrogen and progesterone will be in circulation.

SO WHAT HAPPENS AT THE MENOPAUSE?

When the first intimations of the menopause are experienced, they often bring with them a set of new symptoms that have never been experienced before. The menopause may well coincide with a number of other health factors, and the degree of severity may well be associated with the timing of the symptoms and whether you have had a hysterectomy.

TIMING

There is a substantial variation in the timing of the menopause. For the majority of women their last natural period will be somewhere between the ages of 45 and 55, with an average in the UK of 50.78 years, compared with the average onset in the US which is currently 49.8 years. Interestingly, there has been little change in the time of the onset of symptoms over the last hundred years and, even in the Middle Ages, 50 years was about the norm. Age at the onset of the menopause varies between cultures. Black women, for example, tend to experience an earlier menopause than white women in the US, and it can be nearly 10 years earlier in malnourished women from developing countries. Nutrition, chronic infection and chronic illness in developing countries are factors that need to be taken into consideration.

Just why is there such a divergence in the Western population? Several studies have been conducted to find out what determines the age of the menopause. By far the biggest determinant of an early menopause is **smoking**: the more you smoke, the sooner your periods cease. This looks like a toxic effect of something in cigarettes and is yet another reason to stop or cut down if one were needed. Heavy smokers can reach the menopause two years earlier than their non-smoking counterparts.

Other factors that have been linked to a slightly earlier menopause are never having had children, possibly being short or underweight and possibly finishing your last pregnancy before the age of 28. These effects appear small.

Just because your periods begin early does not mean that you will escape your periods earlier. It was once thought that an early start to periods meant that the menopause would be later, but this theory has been discounted.

As the cessation of menstruation is mainly determined by the ovaries running out of eggs, it would not be surprising if the factors present at the time your eggs were being formed are relevant. As this takes place before you were born, perhaps what was going on during your mother's pregnancy needs to be considered. Astonishingly, when the ovaries are developing, some five to seven million follicles are formed by the fifth month of pregnancy. By the time the baby is born this has fallen to around two million and continues to fall thereafter. Mother Nature is already sorting out the wheat from the chaff.

It is now known that the female offspring of smokers are more likely to have difficulty getting pregnant, perhaps because their ovaries have taken a knock. Low birth-weight, being premature or severe illness of the mother during pregnancy might also be factors. We will have to see what future research reveals. Nutrition may well be found to be a factor, too, as smoking adversely affects the levels of many nutrients. Smokers tend to eat less well than non-smokers and, as we shall see, a number of essential nutrients influence hormone metabolism, hormone problems and the function of the ovaries.

The story doesn't end there. During the perimenopause, the run-up to the last actual period, the rate of follicle loss increases in line with the rise in the level of pituitary hormones. It might just be possible for anything that increases the sensitivity of the ovary to respond to these stimulating hormones, such as the balance of certain nutrients, would help to delay the final day. For more information refer to Chapter 7: Nutrition and Hormone Function.

Finally, there are a few unfortunate women who will experience the menopause at a young age, before they are 40. Most but not all of these women have run out of eggs, sometimes naturally, or because they have received anti-cancer drugs or radiotherapy. However, we should not underestimate the possible influence of nutrition from birth to the menopause. If cessation of smoking and a long-term improvement in diet could delay the menopause by three or four years, these women would not have to take HRT for such a long period of time and would therefore be less exposed to some of the long-term delayed risks, especially that of breast cancer.

" Jill's Story "

Jill was only 36 when she began an early menopause. She was on HRT for several years, but eventually the side-effects became too great and she had to come off it. She is a health visitor and counsellor from Leicestershire, with three children. She first approached the WNAS for help seven years ago, at the age of 47.

'In 1976 we were living in Zimbabwe. I was 36 and my children were aged eight, five and two. When I first missed a period my first thought was – was I pregnant again? I didn't feel pregnant, but I saw my doctor and had a pregnancy test which was negative. Nobody was unduly concerned, although I had always had a regular menstrual cycle, so I kept thinking it would come soon. But it didn't.

My doctor referred me to a gynaecologist, who went through my case history and checked my thyroid levels, and then pronounced that he thought I was going through an early menopause. By this time I had missed five periods. He asked me to keep a temperature chart and, lo and behold, I suddenly ran a high temperature and experienced abdominal pain, which was followed by a period. My response was to think: that proves him wrong – fancy suggesting a menopause!

At about this time we were making arrangements to return to England, and there was a lot of stress to deal with: the move, sorting out our house which had been let while we were away, and had gone to rack and ruin in five years, and the fact that my husband was starting his new job and working all hours, including weekends. To crown it all I injured my neck carrying my youngest child in a heavy rainstorm. I was subsequently in agony and unable to sleep.

My doctor prescribed a course of iron tablets for my absent periods, which had not returned, but these did nothing. I remember seeing him one day and saying tearfully that something needed doing, otherwise I felt my marriage would be heading for divorce. I seemed to be constantly tired and irritable, I was getting headaches, felt anxious, my memory wasn't so good and sometimes I felt quite confused. I found it difficult to concentrate and was feeling very low.

I was referred to a consultant who, after doing various tests, said that my ovaries were not functioning. He prescribed HRT, which I had never heard of until then, and I remember feeling very lucky to live near one of the only HRT prescribers in the county at the time. Within days of commencing Cycloprogynova I began to feel like a new person, like my old self again, with the sense of humour I hadn't realised I'd lost! Also I could sleep, and the pain in my neck and the numbness in my arms I had been experiencing went too.

As the weeks and months went by, I found a pattern emerging. There would be approximately 16 days when I felt great, then I began to feel edgy and sailed into a week of PMS symptoms. At the HRT clinic I was prescribed vitamin B6, and also Premarin to take the week I was off the Cycloprogynova. I was also prescribed Moduretic, to deal with the fluid retention. As I had insomnia again during my bad week, my GP also prescribed Halcion.

In March 1985 I read a piece in The Times – "Diet could End Women's Bad Days". It was a report on the research conducted by the WNAS. I wrote for some information which I found very interesting, and I passed it on to my health visitor colleagues and also to my clients. Looking back, I do not know why I didn't ask for some help for myself at that point.

The next 18 months became increasingly stressful. My husband had to take early retirement because of government cuts. We seemed to have endless marital crises, which he blamed on me and my problems. My GP prescribed Diazepam to help relax me during my bad week, which was when things got really out of hand.

I finally phoned the WNAS for myself and spoke to a very reassuring person. She sent me some questionnaires which I duly completed and returned, and a programme was worked out for me to follow. I changed my diet, which I had previously thought was very healthy, took supplements and increased my exercise regime.

Within three months most of my symptoms had gone and I was able to reduce or omit most of the medication I had been taking, but I did continue with the HRT. I carried on, and within six months all my symptoms had gone.

The following summer I developed an odd rash on my legs, like lots of little blood blisters. Because we were not sure of the cause, my GP suggested I come off the HRT for a month. My husband had just been posted abroad, and as the whole family was about to join him for nearly two months, I would have plenty of time to relax, so I thought it would be a good time to try coming off the HRT. I felt fine off the HRT this time, despite the fact that the trip was very stressful, and my relationship with my husband was at breaking point. He refused to communicate or spend any time with me alone, without the children. But, amid all the stress, I still felt more "myself"; I had no desire to be back on the HRT and felt I could cope.

So I came off the HRT finally in May 1988 and haven't taken it since. I mostly observe the WNAS dietary recommendations, still avoiding caffeine, whole wheat and chocolate. I usually manage very well by eating Ryvita and drinking small amounts of decaffeinated coffee. I find that whenever I lapse to any great extent, I start getting digestive problems, can feel very tired and sometimes feel anxious, irritable and moody.

Sadly, I came to recognise the total futility of trying to work at any sort of positive relationship within my marriage and in 1990 I obtained a divorce. I coped with the stress of the breakdown in my marriage, the divorce, having to move house, my father developing senile dementia, three bereavements in the family, financial worries and other problems. I have built a new life for myself and feel happier, more confident and in fact am healthier now than I think I have ever been. Also I now look and feel 10 years younger than I did 10 years ago.'

PMS Symptom Questionnaire

JILL

Symptoms	Week after period (Fill in 3 days after period)				Week before period (Fill in 2–3 days before period)			
	None	Mild	Moderate	Severe	None	Mild	Moderate	Severe
PMT-A					*variable depending on stress factors*			
Nervous tension	✓					✓		
Mood swings	✓						✓	✓ →
Irritability	✓						✓	
Anxiety	✓					✓		
PMT-B								
*Weight gain	✓							
Swelling of extremities	✓						✓ legs	
Breast tenderness	✓					✓		
Abdominal bloating	✓					✓		
PMT-C								
Headache	✓				sometimes	✓		
Craving for sweets	✓					✓		
Increased appetite	✓					✓		
Heart pounding	✓				✓			
Fatigue	✓						✓	✓ →
Dizziness or fainting	✓				✓ (during teens)			

37

PMT-D							
Depression	✓			✓✓	↑	✓	
Forgetfulness	✓		✓✓	✓		✓	
Crying	✓						
Confusion	✓			✓	↑	✓	
Insomnia	✓			✓			

OTHER SYMPTOMS							
Loss of sexual interest	✓						
Disorientation	✓		✓✓	✓			
Clumsiness	✓						
Tremors/shakes	✓		✓✓				
Thoughts of suicide	✓		✓				
Agoraphobia	✓	✓					
Increased physical activity	✓						
Heavy/aching legs	✓		✓✓	✓			
Generalised aches	✓		✓✓				
Bad breath	✓				✓		
Sensitivity to music/light	✓						
Excessive thirst	✓			✓ sometimes			

Do you have any other PRE-MENSTRUAL SYMPTOMS not listed above

1 _____   4 _____

2 _____   5 How much weight do you gain before your period

3 _____   3–4 lbs

Follow-up Menopause Questionnaire

Do you suffer from any of the following? Please ensure each symptom is only ticked *once*.

JILL	* How many times per month	None	Mild	Moderate	Severe
1 Hot/cold flushes*		✓			
2 Facial/body flushing*		✓			
3 Nightsweats*		✓			
4 Palpitations*		✓			
5 Panic attacks*		✓			
6 Generalised aches and pains		✓			
7 Depression		✓			
8 Perspiration		✓			
9 Numbness/skin tingling in arms and legs		✓			
10 Headaches			✓		
11 Backaches			✓		
12 Fatigue		✓			
13 Irritability			✓		
14 Anxiety			✓		
15 Nervousness		✓			
16 Loss of confidence		✓			
17 Insomnia		✓			
18 Giddiness/dizziness		✓			
19 Difficulty/frequency in passing water		✓			
20 Water retention		✓			

21 Bloated abdomen	✓				
22 Constipation	✓				
23 Itchy vagina	✓				
24 Dry vagina	✓				
25 Painful intercourse	✓				
26 Decreased sex drive	✓				
27 Loss of concentration	✓				
28 Confusion/Loss of vitality	✓				

Are any of the above symptoms cyclic? (i.e. come in cycles, for example on a monthly basis) _No ~ they were due to stress at work and in my personal life at the time._

THE PERIMENOPAUSE

You may not have realised that there is another phase in your life that comes before the menopause, known as the perimenopause. *Peri* simply means *around*, and it seems the changes that occur during the perimenopause can begin from anything up to five years before the menopause strikes.

For most women, ovulation is a regular event between the ages of 20 and 40. From approximately the age of 40 onwards, the supply of Graafian follicles begins to run out. There may be cycles in which the level of oestrogen is slightly reduced. The pituitary senses this and increases its release of FSH to stimulate the tiring ovary more slowly, so that the time between cycles becomes longer and shorter. Progesterone levels will fall as ovulation does not always occur.

The second hormone from the pituitary gland, LH, also rises a little later on. As oestrogen levels fall, the lining of the womb loses its main source of stimulation and periods cease. Levels of FSH and LH remain high for several years, as they continue to live in hope, before they finally get the message and subsequently fall away.

Most of us are unprepared for the perimenopause. For some it simply brings a degree of unpredictability into our lives, during which time we experience irregular periods, some may be lighter, while others are heavier, with perhaps the odd hot flush or night sweat. Mood swings often occur and a degree of depression is common. Those least fortunate women may experience a worsening of their PMS symptoms at this time, as well as constant mood swings and more black days than they care to count.

66 Melanie's Story 99

Melanie, a 39-year-old mother of three from Hertfordshire, contacted the WNAS after reading the first edition of this book, *Beat the Menopause Without HRT*.

'My menopause started early at the age of 37, and I was determined not to take HRT or other medication. Having my own business and coping with the menopause at the same time as working long hours was taking its toll. Losing control over my emotions and not being able to deal with everyday normal stresses was affecting my standard of work and relationship with family and friends. I knew I couldn't put up with this for much longer.

The last straw for me was when I contacted my GP when I was feeling really low with various symptoms: no energy, asthma, hayfever and constantly being emotional and depressed. My doctor suggested that unless I took a course of Prozac, he couldn't help me! I knew that this was not the treatment I needed, and was determined to overcome my symptoms naturally with nutrition.

I tried various self-help remedies, but after two years of not really getting anywhere, I read the first edition of this book, Beat the Menopause Without HRT by Maryon Stewart which was really enlightening. After reading the book, my symptoms seemed to make sense, but it occurred to me that actually seeing someone would keep me on the straight and narrow!

An appointment for a consultation with Maryon Stewart in London was arranged. Dietary modifications were recommended as well as a list of supplements to help combat my symptoms. Maryon explained that wheat in the form of bread, cakes and pasta, and caffeine can exacerbate flushes and sweats, so alternatives were suggested. I enjoyed finding new ingredients in the health-food shop and rice cakes soon became a staple part of my diet!

My progress was not as rapid as I had hoped, and after further reading realised that food intolerances were partly to blame. Maryon recommended that I avoid yeast products and all dairy products which really made a difference. My energy levels dramatically increased and this had a positive effect on running the business. It was difficult sticking to such a rigorous diet because I was surrounded by "normal" food and the rest of the family were able to eat bread, cheese and milk quite happily! However, I was determined not to give in because steady weight loss was evident.

I couldn't believe the transformation in my health. My hair was far softer and silky and generally I felt five years younger! My husband was so supportive throughout the programme and as a "reward" he booked surprise tickets to Canada for my cousin's wedding. It was a wonderful experience visiting my family, but I would never have imagined undertaking such a journey before contacting the WNAS!'

WHEN PMS MEETS THE MENOPAUSE

It's pretty bad luck if your premenstrual syndrome bumps into the start of your menopause symptoms, and you have the worst of both worlds. It is a common problem, but fortunately one that can be sorted out effectively within the space of a few months. Numerous studies reveal that the occurrence of cyclical physical and mental symptoms that are present just before the arrival of menstruation and diminish or disappear with or shortly after its arrival are at their most prevalent in the mid-30 age group. So what are they doing here in a book on the menopause? Well, for some women, PMS never quite goes away and can even be worse in the perimenopausal phase. This is presumably due to the hormonal instability at this time. This and other hormone-related factors have caused many researchers in the past to attribute PMS to a lack or an excess of any hormone you care to mention. The medical profession do not speak with one voice in this matter. More critical research, however, has found no consistent hormonal abnormality in the majority of PMS sufferers and a more modern understanding is to ascribe the cause of PMS to an undue sensitivity on the part of the sufferer to the normal hormonal changes that take place in the last half of the cycle. Now this makes it a lot easier to see how PMS might fit in with some women's perimenopausal experience.

Most women who suffer from PMS do not enjoy the hormonal roller-coaster. Furthermore, the most successful treatments include anything that effectively switches off the ovaries. No working ovaries means no PMS! Oestrogen implants work like magic, producing a near-religious experience for some women. But alas, the benefit may not last as the body adjusts to a new hormonal balance and the natural cycle re-imposes itself.

Our own substantial experience and that of others who have also published their results is that PMS can be helped by a change of diet, the use of certain nutritional supplements, and physical exercise. These factors can all influence female hormone chemistry, nervous-system chemistry, general well-being and physical fitness. They can do so in a far more gentle yet as effective a way as the 'best' hormonal treatment.

In our survey mentioned in Chapter 1 we also looked at the relationship between previous PMS suffering and current menopausal symptoms. The difficulty with this sort of question is that the person's perception of the past may be influenced by their current state of health.

There did seem to be a moderate connection between the severity of past premenstrual symptoms and some current menopausal symptoms. This held true for symptoms of depression, anxiety, confusion and insomnia in particular. Physical symptoms, such as hot flushes and night sweats showed only a minor degree of association with past PMS.

It would therefore seem that symptoms that are mainly attributable to oestrogen withdrawal, such as hot flushes, are not greatly influenced by a history of PMS. 'Mental' symptoms, however, do seem to show some kind of continuity. It is not possible from the questions we asked to discern how much of this was due to psychological problems, or hormonal or other health problems.

As diet and lifestyle seem to make such a big difference to many women's PMS, there seems to be hope for many menopausal women suffering with similar mood changes at the time of the menopause.

❝ Annabelle's Story ❞

Annabelle, a florist from Hertfordshire with three grown-up children, was 47 when she approached the WNAS for help. Her PMS symptoms had reached a crescendo, as her menopause symptoms were beginning.

'My periods had gradually become very heavy, leaving me feeling exhausted. During the run-up to each period I felt extremely anxious and irritable, with incredibly sore breasts, having gained about half a stone in weight, which felt like half a ton around my middle.

I thought this was bad enough. Then one day I began having hot flushes and nightsweats as well. My head would throb continually and my heart would pound, and I honestly thought I was going insane. I was so relieved to hear about the WNAS and, apart from anything else, I discovered I was addicted to caffeine. I made dietary changes, which incidentally I had to follow closely, otherwise I fell behind again, and I began an exercise programme, which I felt much better for, and took specific nutritional supplements.

Within a couple of months I was like a different person. All my PMS symptoms had disappeared, the flushes and sweats had gone, and I felt human again. I can honestly say life is normal again and I feel as if the storm is over. I have even managed a three-month trip with my husband to visit our daughter in Australia. I feel reborn.'

Further information on the treatment of PMS and the experience we have had in treating the women attending the Women's Nutritional Advisory Service's clinics can be found in the book *No More PMS!* That said, there will be some women in the perimenopause with premenstrual symptoms who will benefit from some form of hormonal therapy. For them a small dose of HRT in the form of tablet or patch will help smooth out the hormonal swings. Those women with a uterus will need to take a cyclical dose of progesterone and this is associated with a return of PMS symptoms in 20–30 per cent.

If you have some premenstrual symptoms, are in the perimenopause and are undecided about HRT, then read on. PMS is only one factor to consider in deciding how best to control the symptoms of the change.

THE NORMAL MENOPAUSE

The last actual period denotes the date of the menopause itself. This can only be determined with hindsight, usually after there have been no periods for at least six months in a woman of suitable age, with typical symptoms or with hormonal evidence of the menopause. The commonest test is to measure FH, LH and oestrogen levels in the blood.

During the run-up to the menopause there is considerable instability, with all these hormonal changes occurring. Not surprisingly, this is the time when symptoms can be most troublesome, especially if you are already a sufferer of premenstrual syndrome.

〝 Laura's Story 〞

Laura, 41, a previous WNAS PMS patient, lives with her husband in Berkshire. She decided to get in touch with the WNAS because she had improved so much on the PMS programme when she contacted us in 1992. The main thing that prompted Laura to get in touch with us again was that her husband told her she was very difficult to live with as she was so moody.

'I went to my GP for a blood test which showed that I wasn't yet menopausal but I had falling hormonal levels which were causing my symptoms. He said I was "perimenopausal" which is the stage just before starting the menopause. My main problems were flushes, nausea, extreme tiredness and loss of confidence. I benefited so much from the PMS programme that I was inspired to finally get my menopausal symptoms sorted out.

I followed the dietary recommendations which were not dissimilar to the

PMS dietary programme. I had reverted to eating wheat so the first thing I was told to do was to exclude bread, biscuits and pasta. At least this time I was prepared, so making the changes did not come as such as shock. The only main difference was having to include phytoestrogens in my diet. This meant that I used soy milk in place of cow's milk and pulses, but as I am a vegetarian, this was not too difficult.

Three months later I had my second consultation and my symptoms were hardly noticeable; those that had not totally disappeared had been drastically reduced. The added bonus was that I lost 9lbs – thank you, WNAS.'

HYSTERECTOMY

Hysterectomy is the surgical removal of the womb and is one of the commonest operations performed in the UK. Some 20,000 take place here each year and a staggering 590,000 are performed each year in the USA. It involves the removal of the womb, either through an incision in the abdomen or, in about 25 per cent of cases, by it being removed through the vagina. A total hysterectomy just removes the womb including the cervix or neck of the womb. Sometimes the ovaries, which are at either side of the uterus, are also removed together with neighbouring tissues; this is called a radical hysterectomy. The ovaries may need to be removed if they are diseased with large cysts, endometriosis or cancer.

Studies have revealed a great variation in the number of hysterectomies performed, especially in different regions of the USA. Although there is agreement about the need for hysterectomy in women with uterine cancer, there is not much agreement about its need when the reasons are non-cancerous, such as fibroids, heavy periods and pelvic pain. Recently, two detailed American publications have looked at why hysterectomies are performed and their outcome. Data collected by the National Center for Health Statistics in Atlanta revealed that just under 600,000 hysterectomies were performed per year for the years 1988–90. The overall rate per year was just below six hysterectomies for every thousand women rising to 10 in the 30 to 54 years age group. The overall rate was slightly higher in black women than white. The commonest reason was uterine fibroids, followed by endometriosis, prolapse and cancer among others. Fibroids were listed as the reason twice as commonly in whites as blacks. The ovaries were removed in 50 per cent of the operations and this became more likely with increasing age. However, oophorectomy, the medical term for the removal of the ovaries, was still performed in 29 per cent of the youngest age group listed, the 25 to 34 years category. For virtually all of these, HRT will be necessary.

The outcomes of 418 hysterectomies were assessed in the second study from the Massachusetts General Hospital. For those women who had the operation because of fibroids, abnormal bleeding or pelvic pain, the outcome was frequently favourable. New problems arose in some with hot flushes (13 per cent), weight gain (12 per cent), depression (eight per cent) and lack of interest in sex (seven per cent) being recorded one year after the operation in those who were not troubled by these problems before it.

Hot flushes were, as you would expect, more likely in those who had had an oophorectomy (14 per cent) but still occurred in three per cent of those whose ovaries were not lost. On a more positive note, only three per cent of women still had negative feelings about themselves as women one year after the operation.

It seems that many women will continue to enter the menopause after having had a hysterectomy with loss of their ovaries. HRT will be offered and taken by a majority of these women, especially in the USA. Those women who have had a hysterectomy because of uterine cancer will not be able to take HRT. This may change if future research shows that HRT is safe in those women in whom the cancer has not returned.

« Carol's Story »

Carol, a 51-year-old mother of two and full-time property surveyor from Yorkshire contacted the WNAS with menopausal symptoms and she was also concerned about her weight and digestion.

'I had a hysterectomy at the age of 37 because of an abscess on my ovaries and endometriosis, and I am now left with only half of one ovary. At the age of 45 when my menopausal symptoms "kicked in", my GP convinced me that it was necessary to take HRT to protect my bones against osteoporosis. When I approached the WNAS I was still taking HRT but wanted to combine it with natural treatment so I could eventually withdraw from the HRT. The main side-effect from HRT was severe water retention which was making me feel bloated and lethargic.

I was sent a comprehensive menopause questionnaire and diet diary which I completed and returned for assessment. The quick response from the

WNAS was impressive and they arranged a telephone consultation for me within two weeks. The telephone service was very efficient, and convenient, too. Questions were asked relating to my background and I had the opportunity to talk freely, asking questions and discussing my problems. To be honest, I was a little apprehensive about speaking to someone over the telephone, but the consultant made me feel at ease and she had so much time for me.

A dietary programme was worked out which recommended that I avoid all wheat, oats, barley and rye for an initial six weeks which would ease the digestive problems and encourage steady weight loss. It was explained that sometimes weight loss can be difficult if you are eating foods to which you are sensitive, at the same time encouraging fluid retention. Because I was relying on HRT for my oestrogen, which would stop if it was discontinued, I was told to eat plenty of naturally occurring plant oestrogens which work in a similar way to the natural form produced by your body. By doing so, it would also reduce the risk of breast cancer and osteoporosis.

The diet was easy to follow because I already ate healthily, trying to incorporate as many "hormone-friendly" foods each day. I would start the day with a "Zest for Life" muesli, which contained lots of nuts and seeds without the wheat, with soy milk, followed by oily fish and salad for lunch, lean meat or fish with fresh vegetables for dinner. The diet was great, and a real bonus for me was weight loss and decreased digestive problems. Cutting out the wheat had drastically alleviated my constipation.

Three months into the programme I had lost over one stone, but it was obvious that if I ate oats and wheat the pounds would creep back on. Most diets that I had followed had been unsuccessful because by the end I became so preoccupied with food that I would give in. The WNAS programme emphasised that it wasn't a "diet" but more a healthy eating plan in tune with my own body's requirements. I don't think I was eating any less on the programme, just excluding certain foods.

I feel confident that the HRT can be discontinued fairly soon because I know that natural alternatives are effective, easy to implement and safe.'

❝ Sarah's Story ❞

Sarah, who lives in Essex, was in her early fifties when she contacted the WNAS for help. She had previously had a hysterectomy and was using Estraderm patches.

'I started my menopause when I was 45. My periods became irregular and extremely heavy. I experienced night shivers which were followed by hot flushes, and disturbed sleep, waking every two hours with tingling limbs. As a result I felt constantly tired and intolerant to others during the daytime. I also had a bloated tummy and evening flushes, which made me uninterested in travel or evening outings in particular.

Although my doctor had prescribed Estraderm patches, I read about the WNAS programme in a magazine and decided to contact them for some additional advice. I found the programme written for me reassuring and experienced some instant benefit, gradually feeling less fatigued. I have continued to avoid red meat, spirits and fried foods.

I am 60 years old now and I still feel great. I'm full of energy and I sleep well. I look forward to each day, meeting friends, going away and returning home. After a good night's sleep I am more tolerant generally and cope far better with my semi-invalid husband. As a result of following the WNAS programme I am now more able to enjoy living instead of it being an effort to get through each day.'

CONTRACEPTION AND THE MENOPAUSE

Women over 40 do get pregnant, and though fertility certainly declines from the late thirties onward, contraception is still an important issue for the perimenopausal woman. A study of older women between the ages of 40 and 55 who were menstruating regularly found that 93 per cent were still ovulating. At the age of 45 the rate of pregnancy is still 10 to 20 per cent of women per year. Hence the need for contraception.

Barrier methods are often the choice. More mature couples may be prepared to use condoms, the diaphragm or contraceptive sponge and foam. The intra-uterine contraceptive device, the coil, may be suitable. Infection and rejection may not be as problematic they are in younger women but heavy periods that worsen will mean that the coil will need to be removed.

Perhaps no contraception is necessary? No period for a year in a woman aged over 50, and for two years in a woman aged 45 to 50, makes pregnancy unlikely but not impossible. If ovulation can be influenced and sustained by an improvement in diet, then be warned! Oral contraception is still possible for the perimenopausal woman who is not looking to increase the size of her family. HRT, it must be remembered, is not an effective contraceptive, as the dosage of oestrogen is not great enough to inhibit natural ovulation should it occur.

There are two different types of oral contraceptive: the combined (oestrogen and progestogen) oral contraceptive (COC), and the progestogen-only pill (POP). Progestogen is the name for synthetic progesterones of which there are several types; these are also used in some HRT preparations to produce a regular withdrawal bleed. COCs can now be given to women of any age provided they are healthy non-smokers with no reason to avoid oestrogen. As the oestrogen in COCs is synthetic, and many times more potent than natural oestrogens, there has to be a greater degree of caution with its use than with that in HRT. COCs cannot be given if there is a history of or the presence of most types of heart disease, a history of blood clots, sickle cell anaemia, most types of liver disease, breast and gynaecological cancers and many rare but serious conditions that were worsened during pregnancy. Particular care needs to be taken with those who have other medical problems or are taking a variety of drugs.

The advantage of COCs in the perimenopause is that they will help to control irregular cycles, they will reduce the symptoms of oestrogen withdrawal and they can minimise bone loss. However, side-effects include breast enlargement, fluid retention, an increase in blood pressure, leg cramps and pains, depression, loss of libido, headaches, weight gain, nausea, patches of increased skin pigmentation, vaginal discharge, cervical erosion and breakthrough bleeding. So it is very much up to each individual to decide whether the possible disadvantages outweigh the benefits.

The large variability in tolerance of the oestrogen-containing oral contraceptives has encouraged interest in the progestogen-only pill, POP. Here, a small dose of a progestogen is taken every day throughout the cycle, even when bleeding occurs. Progestogens may stop ovulation but they also thicken cervical mucus and inhibit implantation of a fertilised egg. They do not stop the hormonal changes of the menopause and do not diminish the symptoms of oestrogen withdrawal. In fact, they could aggravate such symptoms. Their advantage is that they are safer than COCs and are particularly suitable for those who cannot take COCs, especially smokers. Again, POPs cannot be taken by those with a history of severe heart disease, circulation problems and blood clots, those with a history of ectopic pregnancy and in a few other rare situations. They interact with several drugs and special care is needed when they are taken by those with high blood pressure, severe migraine and ovarian cysts. Side-effects are not too common except for irregular bleeding. Breast discomfort, acne, ovarian cysts and headaches can still occur and some women experience depression and haemorrhoids.

So there are the choices. The short- to mid-term risks of these oral contraceptives, provided you can take them, are not great but the full magnitude of the long-term risk will not be apparent until a large number of women in their forties have been using oral contraceptives for 10 years or more. And what will be the risk for these women of then undergoing HRT? Again, the answers will not be known for many years.

For most women in the 40-plus age group who need contraceptive advice, it is worth seeking expert advice from a family-planning counsellor, practice nurse or general practitioner with special interests in these problems. Do bear in mind that if your menopause begins before you are 50 you will need to use contraception for at least two years following your last period, and after 50 it's still contraception for a year, please!

AFTER THE MENOPAUSE

By now you might think that a woman's hormones have left the equivalent of the Garden of Eden to enter the Wilderness. But where there is life, there is hope!

Levels of oestrogen and other hormones do not fall away to nothing. Small but significant amounts of oestrogen are produced by the conversion of normal amounts of androgens (male sex hormones) that are still circulating in the bloodstream. These are produced by the adrenal glands, near the kidneys, and from the remaining part of the ovary. They are then converted into weak oestrogen hormones by chemical reactions in fat tissue, the skin and the adrenal glands themselves. Although these levels are low, they are not insignificant.

Postmenopausal women who develop cancer of the lining of the womb have relatively high levels of oestrogen circulating in their body. As you can imagine, the more fat tissues you have, the more of these residual oestrogens can be formed. So obesity is undoubtedly a risk factor for cancer of the uterus.

In the postmenopause, the levels of FSH and LH eventually fall away, and with this stage comes a relatively stable hormonal situation with fewer symptoms but with a greater risk of conditions such as heart disease and osteoporosis. These risks are in part due to the fall in oestrogen and in part due to age, diet and other factors.

IS THE MENOPAUSE PRIMARILY HORMONAL?

The view widely held until recently is that virtually all the symptoms of the menopause could be explained on the basis of a failure by the ovaries. Such a view was strongly supported by the experience and testimony of many women who had undergone HRT and experienced dramatic relief from many or all of their symptoms. While there is indeed a strong relationship between some of the symptoms of the menopause and the falling levels of the hormone oestrogen, because we are extremely complex animals, it stands to reason that there are some other biological mechanisms at play. These should not only be considered but should also open the door to alternative and more natural solutions to HRT, and we will be examining this issue in the last chapter.

3
THE SYMPTOMS OF THE MENOPAUSE

These fall roughly into three groups: physical symptoms, some of which are directly due to the withdrawal of oestrogen, some not so directly, and mental symptoms.

THE SIGNIFICANCE OF OESTROGEN

The main and predominant symptoms that can be attributed to the withdrawal of oestrogen are:

Hot flushes
Nightsweats
Vaginal dryness
Loss of libido
Difficulties with intercourse
Urinary symptoms
Skin changes

Oestrogen acts like all hormones by stimulating a change in certain tissues. It acts predominantly on the tissues of the female reproductive system, the uterus or womb, the vagina, the vulva and the end portion of the urethra – the outlet for the passage of urine from the bladder. Oestrogen also influences breast tissue; it also affects skin tissue and blood vessels, although this does not result in the production of hot flushes.

Hot flushes

Degree of hot flushes in a survey of 500 women

None	Mild	Moderate	Severe	Total suffering
12.5%	23.5%	36%	28%	87.5%

Hot flushes, as they are known in the UK (hot flashes in the USA), are the commonest symptom of the menopause and actually have several components.

In our *Woman's Realm* survey of 500 women, hot flushes were experienced by 87.5 per cent. Other surveys have found that they affect 70–80 per cent of menopausal women. In our survey we also found that they were more likely to be a problem in women who experienced their menopause at a younger age. For these women there is perhaps a more abrupt hormonal change being imposed on a system that has had less time to adapt.

The flush is usually felt over the upper trunk, neck, face and arms. The first event is an increase in blood flow to the affected area of skin. This is followed by redness or a flush, a rise in skin temperature of about 1° Celsius, and then sometimes by sweating which acts to cool the skin. There may be a rise in pulse rate at about the same time as the sensation of heat is experienced, and there can be a small rise in blood pressure. As you would expect with the increase in the flow of blood to the skin and the subsequent sweating, there is loss of heat from the body and a tiny but perceptible drop in the temperature of the inside of the body. At the time of or just before the flush there are some changes in the levels of certain hormones – but not in the level of oestrogen!

The flush is preceded by a surge in hormone activity, not by the pituitary gland, but by an area of the brain called the hypothalamus, adjacent to the pituitary. Many hormones are released including the one that causes a rise in the level of LH from the pituitary. It also appears that there is a surge of activity in the part of the nervous system that controls the adrenal glands, blood pressure and blood flow. Not surprisingly, this is connected to the hypothalamus. So the hot flush is not due to a sudden change in sex hormones but to a change in the activity of that part of the brain that has the main influence over the pituitary. It seems that the pituitary is not the conductor of the hormonal orchestra but the conductor's baton and it is the hypothalamus that is calling the tune. This part of the brain also controls the appetite, the timing of the menstrual cycle and temperature regulation. It appears therefore that the hot flush is as much a 'brain event' as it is a hormonal one.

But what part does oestrogen play?

It appears that these events of the flush only take place if oestrogen has been present in the system and is then withdrawn. Young girls before puberty do not flush, neither do those very few unfortunate girls whose ovaries are unable ever to make oestrogen. They will flush if they are given oestrogen and it is then stopped. Some women on HRT feel better if they can take oestrogen all the time without stopping and starting it, but oestrogen can only be taken continuously if you have had a hysterectomy (because of the risk of cancer of the uterus).

So a hot flush is due to a withdrawal of oestrogen rather than a lack of it. It can even happen when the oestrogen level is high and falling. There is more information about this aspect of the menopause in Chapter 8 which deals with the side-effects of HRT.

Not all women are flushers and women clearly show enormous variability in the degree to which they do flush. Experiments on women who do flush have shown that between hot flushes they experience small but definite irregularities in the flow of blood to the skin of the forearm and that these irregularities are diminished by giving oestrogen. So HRT acts both on the brain and the blood vessels of the skin to combat the hot flush.

Hot flushes, if frequent, greatly affect the quality of life. The flush is strongly associated with sweats in the day or at night. The flushes at night disturb sleep and this may be due to the changes in brain chemistry that precede the flush rather than just the flush itself. Flushers tend to have more menopausal symptoms than non-flushers and these include mental symptoms such as irritability and depression as well as physical symptoms such as aches and pains and tiredness.

Eventually (well, almost always), the system adjusts itself to the withdrawal of oestrogen. This can take months or years. The menopause is really a testing time for many women and the test is in part 'How well can your body chemistry cope with a falling level of oestrogen?' The solution is often just to give oestrogen in some form, but other approaches that help your chemical and nervous system can also be of benefit.

❝ Alison's Story ❞

Alison is a fashion designer from Cheltenham in Gloucestershire. She was 49 when she contacted the WNAS for help with her hot flushes. I remember speaking to her when she had just retired from teaching and was hoping to set up her own business. We decided that the day of her consultation was going to be the first day of the rest of her life in more ways than one.

'When my periods became irregular I assumed my menopause was under way. I didn't seem to have any problems, until the flushes began. The flushes became very severe both during the day and at night. I lived in dread of them, and as their timing was so unpredictable I never knew when one was going to

strike. They made me feel very uncomfortable, especially the cold dampness that remained afterwards. I was unable to get enthusiastic about anything – and I live on my creativity. I just felt stressed, irritable and extremely tired. I used to get at least 12 hot flushes during the day and about eight each night. It was quite exhausting. If I exerted myself even slightly, just by walking up a hill, or experienced the simplest problem at work, I would instantly have a hot flush. And many other flushes came without any apparent reason.

A friend at a yoga class happened to have had similar problems, and was helped by the WNAS. I didn't hesitate to contact them myself and was soon on a new diet, taking special vitamin and mineral supplements and doing more exercise. It took exactly one week for the symptoms to disappear. I was utterly amazed at the speed of recovery. I have not looked back since, except for one or two hiccups the cause of which I can pinpoint. That was a year ago. My friends comment all the time on how much better I look, and my close friends would admit that I'm not crabby any more. It's so nice to be back in control.'

Nightsweats

Degree of nightsweats in a survey of 500 women

None	Mild	Moderate	Severe	Total suffering
25%	18%	32%	25%	75%

Nightsweats commonly accompany hot flushes as they are both due to the same mechanism. In our survey, nightsweats did not seem to tie up with any symptom other than hot flushes. This confirms the concept that they are both due to the withdrawal of oestrogen and that with the other symptoms some other factors apart from hormonal change are at play.

Vaginal dryness

Degree of vaginal dryness in a survey of 500 women

None	Mild	Moderate	Severe	Total suffering
41%	20%	24%	15%	59%

This was very strongly associated with pain on intercourse especially in the slightly older hysterectomised women. It was also associated with loss of libido. It appears that vaginal dryness is a relatively late menopausal problem and this concurs with other research.

The decline in oestrogen results in a decrease in the blood flow to the area, with a loss of elasticity in the tissues and a shrinkage of the cells in the vagina, vulva, uterus, bladder, urethra and breast tissues. Similar but lesser changes also take place in the skin. As a result, the vagina becomes drier and less elastic. These changes can be reversed by the use of oestrogen preparations by mouth or applied in the form of a cream to the vagina and vulva. As we shall see later, oestrogen as HRT is not the only way to promote a return to youthfulness in these tissues. They can also respond to natural oestrogens in our diet.

Oestrogen also influences the nerves that sense touch in the area of the vulva and vagina. Touch perception is obviously important when it comes to sexual arousal and response. The responsiveness of these nerves is reduced as oestrogen levels fall at the menopause but it can be restored to its previous level of sensitivity with the use of HRT. Again it appears that some of the effects of oestrogen are due to its effects on the nervous system and not just on the tissues of the vagina and vulva. Dietary changes, particularly those that include phytoestrols, the plant forms of oestrogen, have also been shown to return the vaginal tissue to normal (see page 189).

The changes in the health and sensitivity of these tissues can obviously influence sexual activity. Vaginal dryness makes intercourse more difficult and, together with a reduction in touch sensitivity, less satisfying. A lessening of interest leads to less intercourse and this increases the rate of change in the vaginal tissues. So it's a bit of a vicious circle!

❝ Iris's Story ❞

Iris was a 52-year-old licensee from Gwent, who had two grown-up children. She had been suffering with menopausal symptoms for a year prior to contacting the WNAS for help.

'I had had an awful year. I had lost my sister from cancer, and had begun my menopause in the space of a few months. My doctor prescribed HRT patches, Prempak, but because of side-effects of severe migraine and considerable weight gain, I was switched to Nuvelle, and then to Prempak-C. I still had awful side-effects and the flushes persisted despite the HRT. I was also suffering with constipation, which made me panic as my sister developed constipation just before her cancer was diagnosed. Plus I had gastric reflux, and although my doctor was very supportive, he had little on offer to eradicate these symptoms.

I read about the WNAS in an article in the Daily Express, *and decided to contact them for help. I followed their advice, and gradually weaned myself off the HRT. Within a month my flushes had calmed down considerably and so had the gastric reflux. The constipation and the wind had gone completely, and my husband was finding it hard to believe how well I seemed.*

I have been following the WNAS recommendations for over a year now, and feel really well. I no longer have a dry vagina, my joints don't ache any more since introducing Efacal into my programme, and unless I am very stressed both my menopause symptoms and my gastric reflux are memories only. I really enjoy the diet, and feel so much better generally for the exercise and regular relaxation.'

Loss of libido

Degree of loss of libido in a survey of 500 women

None	Mild	Moderate	Severe	Total suffering
38%	18%	21%	23%	62%

This, not surprisingly, was associated with vaginal dryness especially in those who had had a hysterectomy. Pain on intercourse was not a very strongly associated symptom. Anxiety, insomnia and even aches and pains were all mildly associated with loss of sexual interest. So what does this all mean? It looks as though there is a mixture of factors at work. Loss of libido in this group did not have the pattern we would expect if it were a straightforward 'hormone-deficiency' problem as some experts argue. Nor did it have the characteristics of being a predominantly psychological problem. It would seem to vary from person to person with some influence due to hormonal change causing vaginal dryness.

66 Diane's Story 99

Diane is a 50-year-old wife, mother and carer from Aberdare in Wales. When she approached the WNAS for help she had been suffering with her symptoms for seven years.

'I was still working full-time in the education department of our local government office. The first menopausal symptom I experienced was that I found it harder and harder to concentrate. This in turn led to a lack of self-confidence which affected my performance at work and my life at home.

I had to take time off and get others to stand in for me, as jobs that should have taken five minutes were taking hours. I even apologised to my boss for my incompetence and told him that I was thinking of resigning. I had always loved my career, but for the first time in my life I was thinking of giving it up.

I then started to feel constantly ill with migraine headaches and hot flushes. I felt that I had hit rock-bottom emotionally. I felt haggard and undesirable. I seemed to have aged almost overnight.

My husband had always been very supportive but my irrational behaviour and my loss of libido were putting quite a strain on our relationship. I knew my behaviour wasn't fair to anyone, including myself, so I went to see my doctor and was given a prescription for antidepressants. They didn't work and made me feel that not only was I experiencing menopausal symptoms, but also that I was mentally ill. Still feeling low I saw another doctor, who this time prescribed HRT.

For six months I felt on top of the world. Most of my symptoms disappeared, although my libido didn't fully recover. Then the migraines returned with a vengeance and once again I couldn't sleep and was feeling sick and suffering with diarrhoea. My legs felt like lead; in fact I had no energy at all and found it an effort to walk. Plus I had terrible sugar cravings. I felt as if I was back to square one. I actually took myself off HRT and contacted the Women's Nutritional Advisory Service for help.

I was instructed to make specific dietary changes, took nutritional supplements and exercised regularly. The hot flushes stopped within two weeks. My migraine headaches lifted completely and within a short time my whole attitude to life became more positive. From lying in bed feeling depressed, I noticed that come the morning I wanted to jump out of bed and get on with the day, just like I had when I was younger. Once again I had lots of energy, my moods were much more constant and I no longer felt irrational. Thankfully my libido returned and a normal loving relationship with my husband was resumed. I felt much more confident and even the laughter lines on my face noticeably faded.

It's been four years now and I still feel absolutely brilliant. I am delighted with my progress and feel as if I have been released from a prison. My husband is very relieved too as he felt so helpless at the time. Within six months I was a totally different person and I have never looked back. I need far less sleep now. I'm planning to take an Open University degree course and I'm learning to play the piano. I feel tremendous, like a new woman, and best of all I look like one, too.'

Difficulties with intercourse

Degree of pain on intercourse in a survey of 500 women

None	Mild	Moderate	Severe	Total suffering
64%	15%	12%	9%	36%

As we have already seen, this was mainly associated with vaginal dryness especially in older, non-hysterectomised women.

Urinary symptoms

Although we didn't ask about these in our survey, they do deserve a mention as they can sometimes be a problem at this time of life.

Loss of control, especially when coughing, laughing or sneezing, an increase in the frequency with which the bladder needs to be emptied during the day or night and a feeling of urgency can all be problems associated with the menopause. It is not clear how much these are due to the fall in oestrogen and how much to the passage of time.

Although urinary symptoms can respond to treatment with HRT, improved control can also be obtained by the use of exercises to improve the muscles around the bladder.

It does appear that some women are also troubled by more frequent urine infections at this time and this is perhaps due to a change in the health of these tissues.

Skin changes

Oestrogens also influence the quality of our skin. The decline in quality at the time of the menopause is associated with thinning of the skin, a reduction in the blood-flow to the skin and a loss of elasticity. These are largely reversed with the use of HRT. Good nutrition and exercise also seem to have a significant influence on skin quality. Those who have very thin skin may also have thin bones. Bones are not just made of minerals: one-third consists of collagen, the main connective tissue of skin. Although some benefit to skin can accrue as a result of HRT it is not known for how long this will last. Perhaps diet and even exercise will become more important with the passage of years.

OTHER PHYSICAL SYMPTOMS OF THE MENOPAUSE

Our survey of 500 women asked about other physical symptoms that can also be a problem around the time of the menopause.

Aches and pains

Severity of aches and pains in a survey of 500 women

None	Mild	Moderate	Severe	Total suffering
29%	19%	32%	20%	71%

Aches and pains have not always been considered part of the menopause and postmenopause. However, some doctors now regard these as a fairly common associated problem that can respond to HRT. But is this really the case?

When we looked at this group of women we found no association between aches and pains and either hot flushes, nightsweats or vaginal dryness. What did come up was that aches and pains were most usually associated with panic attacks in the hysterectomy group and tended to be more of a problem in the younger women in this group. It would seem that many of the women who had had a hysterectomy were not as well as some of their contemporaries. It is not possible to say why, but there could be a dietary rather than a hormonal connection.

For the remaining women who still had their womb, aches and pains were not connected with panic attacks but they were related to insomnia. So it would seem that this could be a reason for some of these women's disturbed sleep.

Again we see that not all women fall into the same category at the time of the menopause, and that the symptoms are not always hormonally related. Clearly, a lot more research and a flexible attitude to the possible causes of these problems is needed before we can say why women are troubled in the way they are at this time of their lives.

« Jeanette's Story »

Jeanette was a 51-year-old mother and post-mistress from Sussex who had been suffering with hot flushes for three years when she contacted the WNAS for advice.

'At the age of 48 my periods came to an end after only slight disruption, and I thought that was that. I had always been quite active and aware of what I ate and drank, and therefore assumed that I had passed through the menopause unscathed.

The hot flushes arrived one day suddenly and took me by surprise. I would get so hot I could smell my hair, and my heart would pound. Then it would subside leaving me shivering, utterly soaked with perspiration. Then the nightsweats began, every night, several times a night, leaving me awake and fretful over the silliest things. I had also become very irritable and short-tempered and constantly tired.

I read an article in Essentials magazine around this time, about the WNAS, which recommended the first edition of this book, Beat the Menopause without HRT. I bought the book and read it, not dreaming for a moment that I would one day become a 'case history' in it! I followed the self-help recommendations, adjusting my eating and drinking habits, and within weeks saw an improvement. Over several months the severe day flushes reduced to milder sweats, the nightsweats continued, but I was sleeping a little better.

I had begun to feel pain in my thumb and finger joints, and they were becoming a little swollen. Pain was also starting in my feet. The pain became more frequent and more severe. I reached a point where holding a pen became almost unbearable. I had watched my mother suffer severely with rheumatoid arthritis, and I found the prospect of suffering similarly a very depressing prospect.

Although I had been following the dietary recommendations, to date I had not taken any supplements, and so decided to contact the WNAS for advice. I went along to my appointment during which time I was given a nutrition and exercise programme and advised on which supplements to take. I mentioned then that I suffered with palpitations, but as I had been having these daily since I was 14, I did not expect that they would be affected by the programme. After only a few weeks the pains in my hands and feet had reduced dramatically and the flushes were slowly vanishing. Three months later I have no pain or swollen joints in my hands or feet, I have no hot flushes day or night, and my palpitations have almost disappeared too, which was something I was sure I would live with for the rest of my life!

I no longer experience the feelings of anxiety I had grown used to, and my family notice that I am much calmer. In addition to all this, my concentration has returned and with it my confidence, which had previously disappeared. I feel that I have been given my old life back and am very grateful.'

Palpitations

Severity of palpitations in a survey of 500 women

None	Mild	Moderate	Severe	Total suffering
47%	24%	23%	6%	53%

Palpitations were not often a severe problem. They were an interesting physical symptom to look at because the different schools of thought could relate them to the hot flushes and the surge of nervous-system activity that accompanies them, or to underlying feelings of anxiety or to the consumption of caffeine from tea and coffee: three quite different possibilities.

Fatigue

This is another common symptom which unfortunately we were unable to ask about because of lack of space on the magazine page. A low energy level is a more common complaint in women than men, and some women report improvement when they take HRT. HRT the elixir of youth? Not quite. A more considered assessment of the cause and treatment of fatigue and other physical symptoms is that if these symptoms are strongly associated with symptoms of oestrogen withdrawal then they may improve with the use of HRT. This has been described as the domino-effect. Well worth having and probably more relevant for the younger woman with more severe hot flushes. As we will see later, and from Philippa's story, HRT is not the only way to control hot flushes and the symptoms of oestrogen withdrawal.

« Philippa's Story »

Philippa is a 45-year-old wife and mother from Reading in Berkshire. She was prescribed HRT by her doctor to help with her menopause symptoms, but was unable to continue as it made her migraine headaches unbearable.

'I had been helped by the WNAS some 12 years ago when I was suffering with severe PMS. With those awful symptoms behind me for years it did not occur to me that I would have a rough menopause.

When my periods became irregular and lighter I suspected that I was starting my menopause. Gradually I became tired, irritable and tearful, with no confidence at all. I visited my doctor to discuss the problem, but he only prescribed antidepressants, which did improve the tearfulness and nausea, but I was still getting the flushes and my vagina had become dry. I was feeling so low by this time I couldn't be bothered to talk to people or make the effort to visit them, which was so unlike me. I couldn't face having anyone to dinner either because of the effort it would take.

I generally felt so tired, drained and tearful, and the worst thing for me was that I didn't have the energy to look after my grandson. I remember sitting on a stool at the kitchen sink after dinner, looking at the dishes that needed clearing away, and wanting to cry because I had not got the energy just to put them in the dishwasher.

I went to visit my doctor again to discuss the possibility of undergoing HRT, which I had read so much about in the media. He wasn't sure if it was suitable as I make breast lumps and have to have regular checks at the hospital. He wanted me to check with the consultant on my next visit. I was so desperate to feel normal again that I wrote to the consultant for the OK!

I was put on Prempak-C at first, but I started to experience intense migraine headaches. I was changed to a lower dose to see whether that made any difference and, finally, I was put on Trisequens. As the migraines persisted I was unable to continue on HRT and that's when I contacted the WNAS for some natural help.

Once again the WNAS formulated a programme for me to follow, this time for my menopause symptoms. I made some dietary changes, took different nutritional supplements and resumed an exercise programme. Within a few months I was feeling better. I have never looked back. My confidence returned. I find myself running up the stairs now, whereas before I felt as if I were climbing a mountain, every stair was such an effort. The nausea has gone. I am much more able to socialise and go to work. I have even taken some courses on computers at an adult college, which I could never have done before. Once again I am delighted with the help of the WNAS.'

Bowel problems

In addition to typical menopausal symptoms we also asked in our survey about bowel problems and how many women suffered from constipation, diarrhoea or both. I knew that women with severe PMS seemed, in nearly 50 per cent of cases, to have bowel problems too, and other surveys have shown that over 20 per cent of the normal adult female population admit to bowel problems.

The pattern of bowel problems in this group was as follows: constipation: 39.5 per cent; diarrhoea: 20 per cent; both: 15.5 per cent. This means that a total of 59.5 per cent of our sample were experiencing bowel problems. Although we cannot relate this to the hormonal changes, it again seems surprisingly high. As there is a known strong connection between diet and bowel problems, these figures would seem to strengthen the need for dietary advice to be given to menopausal women.

Weight-gain following HRT

From our sample, 62 per cent of those who were on HRT claimed that they had experienced weight-gain as a result. The average claimed weight-gain was $16^{1}/_{2}$ pounds. We have no way of accounting for other causes of weight-gain in this survey. Suffice it to say that many women perceive weight-gain as being a problem that goes hand-in-hand with HRT.

MENOPAUSE AND YOUR MIND

Having looked at physical menopausal symptoms, we now come to the 'mental' symptoms of the postmenopause.

Many researchers have already tried to determine if depression, anxiety and insomnia become more of a problem to women as they approach the menopause. The results have been rather mixed, probably because of difficulties in the methods of looking at psychological problems, in relying on subjective reports rather than using standardised tests. This is indeed a criticism of our survey but then we do not wish to rely on our findings alone.

Dr Myra Hunter, a psychologist and the author of *Your Menopause* has developed, together with colleagues, a more scientific method of assessing symptoms. They surveyed 850 women aged 45 to 65 who were not attending a menopause clinic and were thought to be fairly representative of the normal female population of this age. Women around the time of and after the menopause had greater levels of depression and insomnia but not anxiety. The increase in these symptoms was nowhere near as great as the increase in hot flushes. There was no increase in many physical symptoms or in problems related to thinking. The experience of the menopause seemed to make a modest but definite increase in mood changes.

So what pattern did we see in the group of women from *Woman's Realm?*

Insomnia

Degree of insomnia in a survey of 500 women

None	Mild	Moderate	Severe	Total suffering
27%	18%	28%	27%	73%

Clearly a common problem, one as common as hot flushes and nightsweats.

Insomnia was more of a problem in those with anxiety and, to a slightly lesser degree, with nightsweats. Depression and aches and pains also seemed to be mildly associated. So again there could be hormonal, psychological or possibly other physical factors behind insomnia at this time of life. It all depends on the individual.

It is well-documented from other research that insomnia is a common accompaniment of nightsweats. In fact, the disturbance in sleep begins before the sweating does and is in time with subtle changes in the electrical brainwaves, again testimony to the involvement of the nervous system in the symptoms of the menopause.

Anxiety

Degree of anxiety in a survey of 500 women

None	Mild	Moderate	Severe	Total suffering
30%	21%	27%	22%	70%

Panic attacks were strongly associated with those who had had a hysterectomy. Depression was also associated with anxiety and so was insomnia. Here we see quite a strong grouping of different mental complaints. Some would argue that this is good evidence of the need for treatment with drugs to control either the anxiety or depression. Not so fast, we say! With the problems of Valium, Ativan and other benzodiazepine drugs still fresh in our memories there must be another way for the majority of women. We know from our experience of women with premenstrual syndrome that many can do well through dietary change, the use of some nutritional supplements, and physical exercise. Don't jump to conclusions yet.

** Eleanor's Story **

Eleanor is a 43-year-old mother of three from Kent, who had to give up her job at the time her menopause began because she felt so ill.

'Although I was still menstruating at the time, I was feeling so "unwell", constantly exhausted, with loss of memory, an imbalance of mind, headaches, anxiety, panic attacks and rapid mood changes. I felt desperate and quite dreadful, and afraid of being institutionalised.

I was recommended to the WNAS by a friend. I followed a postal and telephone course of treatment which gave me instant hope. It was practical and positive and I felt the benefit almost immediately. Now three years on I am much better. I still avoid caffeine, alcohol and wheat-based products. I am much more balanced and can have normal relationships. Thank God I heard of the wonderful work the WNAS are doing.'

Depression

Severity of depression in a survey of 500 women

None	Mild	Moderate	Severe	Total suffering
31%	23%	30%	16%	69%

As you may well expect, this clusters together with anxiety in the main, and slightly with panic attacks and insomnia, and is in line with what we would expect. But again, don't reach for the happy pills as something a little more natural is to hand.

❝ Moira's Story ❞

Moira is a teacher from Dyfed in Wales who had suffered with menopausal depression for 17 years, at one point so severely she tried to commit suicide. After years of tranquillisers and psychiatric treatment, at the age of 59 she followed the WNAS programme, which changed her life.

'The menopause took me by surprise at the age of 43. I had hot flushes, dizziness and abdominal bloating, but my main symptom was depression, which led to a nervous breakdown. Everything was an effort, even getting up in the morning. I had the feeling I wasn't really there. It was a great disappointment after leading such a full life with a busy and satisfying career.

My husband was very supportive, but at a loss to know how to help me. No-one really understood how I felt. My GP tried different treatments but nothing really helped. Eventually, a psychiatrist gave me mood stabilisers and taught me how to relax. I recovered and returned to my teaching career. However, once I retired the depression got worse and I was just existing. I completely lost confidence and nothing in life seemed to give me any pleasure.

Luckily I read an article which mentioned the Women's Nutritional Advisory Service. After asking me lots of questions and taking a thorough medical history, they worked out a diet, supplement and exercise programme to suit me. Within three weeks I experienced dramatic improvement. During the following four months I had monthly consultations during which adjustments were made to my programme and I felt better than I could remember for many years.

It has been four years since I followed the WNAS programme. I continue to enjoy life now. I'm still symptom-free and I no longer need to take psychiatric *drugs. But I do wish I hadn't left it so late to find effective help. I would like to stress to other women how important it is to get help early on. You do need something other than tablets. So often when you are down you feel powerless to help yourself, and family and friends are at a loss to know how to help. I'm just glad I found the WNAS and can now look to the future with enthusiasm.'*

Confusion

Severity of confusion in a survey of 500 women

None	Mild	Moderate	Severe	Total suffering
39%	24%	26%	11%	61%

Although not that common as a severe symptom, confusion was often marked as a moderate or mild problem. The pattern of its association marked it down as more of a mental symptom than a hormone-related one.

Panic attacks

Severity of panic attacks in a survey of 500 women

None	Mild	Moderate	Severe	Total suffering
47%	22%	21%	10%	53%

Not as common as some other symptoms, the clustering showed that panic attacks mainly tied up with anxiety and depression as well as with aches and pains.

By now a very strong pattern of symptoms is appearing. Those due primarily to the hormonal change of oestrogen withdrawal were clustered together and those that related to anxiety and depression were also clustered together with very little apparent crossover and no age-related influence at the menopause.

It would seem that the full range of menopausally related symptoms cannot be easily explained by the simple notion of 'a lack of hormones'. HRT cannot, therefore, solve all of women's menopausal problems. It would seem that a more broadly based lifestyle approach is needed to give the best chance of success in controlling the troubles of the post-menopause.

PART TWO
THE OESTROGEN FACTOR

4
MEDICAL RISKS FOLLOWING THE MENOPAUSE

The oestrogen circulating around the body prior to the menopause affords the majority of women ongoing protection against a number of serious conditions including heart disease, osteoporosis (the bone-thinning disease) and possibly dementia and even arthritis. However, when oestrogen levels fall at the time of the menopause and beyond, the incidence of these debilitating, and sometimes fatal, conditions escalates significantly. Prior to the menopause, for example, far more men than women become victims of heart disease, whereas post-menopause, the risk for women rises to exceed that of men.

HEART DISEASE

Coronary heart disease is now the most common cause of death of women in Western societies, with heart attacks claiming more than three times more lives than breast cancer and strokes. It actually accounts for 21 per cent of deaths of women over the age of 45 in the UK, and it is estimated that it costs the UK economy in excess of £10 billion each year.

According to research, cardiovascular disease is also the commonest preventable cause of death. There has been little improvement, as yet, in these figures in countries such as the UK and Australia, although the USA and Finland have begun to achieve a substantial fall in their incidence of heart disease. Smoking, lack of exercise, obesity, high blood pressure and high blood cholesterol are all well-documented risk factors and these last three are all influenced by our diet, as you will discover in Chapter 6.

OSTEOPOROSIS

Likewise, osteoporosis, which means 'porous bones' has literally become an epidemic in the Western world, with an estimated five million sufferers in the UK alone. Every three minutes someone in the UK sustains a fracture due to osteoporosis. Approximately 20 per cent of hip-fracture victims die within six months of their accident, with hip fractures claiming more lives than cancer of the ovaries, cervix and uterus combined. The Australians estimate that over 50 per cent of people with hip fractures will require long-term nursing care, which presents an ever-increasing bill as the population ages.

DEMENTIA

Although many of us joke about pre-senile dementia, true dementia is really no joke. One in five elderly people develops dementia, with women being at greater risk post-menopause. Dementia is characterised by a loss of cognition, which means a loss of the ability to function mentally in a variety of ways. Deficiencies may occur in the following areas: memory, use of language, visual awareness of space perception, thinking, problem solving and personality. Significant loss of two or more of these functions would point to dementia.

ARTHRITIS

Both Rheumatoid arthritis and osteoarthritis are common complaints associated with the ageing process. In rheumatoid arthritis, sufferers experience swelling and pain in both small and large joints, which is largely due to inflammation causing an increase in fluid surrounding the joints. Osteoarthritis has quite a different cause. In this type of arthritis there is a loss of the protective surface of cartilage over the ends of bones, with subsequent changes to the underlying bone. This often leads to swelling and distortion of the joints, and most commonly occurs in the joints at the end of the fingers and in the knees.

From the perimenopause onwards, three times as many women as men are likely to suffer with rheumatoid arthritis, with symptoms of stiffness, especially in the morning, often beginning in the winter months. Osteoarthritis affects at least 10 per cent of the over sixties, with women more commonly becoming victims of osteoarthritis in their fingers.

Until relatively recently, conventional doctors have promoted Hormone Replacement Therapy (HRT) as the treatment of choice at the time of the menopause, not only to alleviate symptoms at the time of the menopause, but also to help to prevent this catalogue of unpleasant conditions that await many of us after the menopause. While HRT may be helpful in certain circumstances, like most treatments, it also has weaknesses, as you will discover in the next chapter. Research has progressed to the point where we know that HRT is by no means the only horse in the race either to control menopausal symptoms or to prevent the debilitating conditions outlined above, as you will see in Chapter 9.

5
THE RATIONAL APPROACH TO HORMONE REPLACEMENT THERAPY

Hormone replacement therapy (HRT) has been available in an increasing number of forms for 30 years and numerous studies have been performed to assess the merits and demerits of this treatment. One would have thought that with so many studies over such a long time there should now be a clear general agreement or consensus on its use. However, there are still widely divergent opinions within the medical profession and the consumer certainly does not speak with one voice.

Approximately 75 per cent of women consuming a Western diet will suffer from significant symptoms at the time of the menopause, which means that there are potentially millions of women needing help at this time. HRT is widely promoted as the treatment of choice, but there is much controversy. The consumer is likely to encounter articles that promote HRT either as a new wonder treatment or are scathing about its effects, which is all very confusing. This chapter aims to present both views of HRT so that consumers and potential consumers can make informed choices.

In the United Kingdom a very high percentage of women who commence on HRT discontinue it within the first year, often to the consternation of the family doctor and specialist. Why? Essentially, I don't think that many women quite trust their own doctor's interpretation of the evidence of the benefits and problems associated with HRT usage. This view is supported by the rather conservative attitude that many British academics have towards HRT who, quite rightly, are waiting for the results of further studies designed properly to assess the risks and benefits of HRT, especially in the long term.

GP survey on the menopause

A recent survey of a thousand GPs was carried out in an attempt to assess the help that is currently available for menopausal women. The questions focused on HRT, frequency of its use, side-effects, and incorporation of alternative treatments for the menopause. The survey revealed some interesting and surprising statistics, which are detailed below.

Analysis of the survey revealed that 36 per cent of all women who seek help for the menopause are prescribed HRT. However, 54 per cent of those recommended to take it actually do, and 46 per cent don't, which would indicate a degree of dissatisfaction with the treatment! In fact, according to GPs, 21 per cent of women taking HRT actually come off it within a year, so overall, less than 50 per cent of the women who were advised to take HRT are still taking it.

One question in the survey asked what factors would discourage the doctors from prescribing HRT. The results are detailed in the table below.

	Don't know	Prescribe	Don't Prescribe
Smoking	4%	70%	26%
High blood pressure	2%	90%	8%
Previous history of thrombosis	2%	5%	93
Family history of thrombosis	4%	26%	70%
Pre-existing liver disease	8%	15%	77%
Inactive breast cancer diagnosed in the last five years	4%	5%	91%
Raised cholesterol	8%	75%	17%
Severe migraines	5%	12%	83%

We were particularly surprised that GPs were divided over issues like inactive breast cancer and family history of thrombosis. We were also amazed that so few GPs were concerned about prescribing HRT to women with high blood pressure.

The doctors were asked their opinion on the effectiveness of HRT when prescribed to treat different menopause symptoms and conditions.

	Effective	Not effective	Don't know
Hot flushes	97%	0%	3%
Nightsweats	95%	0%	5%
Vaginal dryness	94%	0%	6%
Fatigue	62%	30%	8%
Depression	55%	36%	9%
Low libido	51%	35%	14%
Aches & pains	44%	41%	15%
Prevention of osteoporosis	91%	0%	9%
Heart disease	65%	11%	21%
Alzheimers	30%	14%	56%

There is clearly a lack of knowledge about the effectiveness of HRT in preventing heart disease and alzheimers. Whilst there is some evidence to support the theory that HRT helps to prevent heart disease, the jury is still out. In fact, at the Third International Symposium on the Role of Soy in Preventing and Treating Chronic Disease (1999), it was broadly agreed that the research on phytoestrogens preventing heart disease was much stronger than the research on HRT and heart disease. As for Alzheimers, the research is still young. There was also a great variation in the number of doctors who use HRT to address fatigue and depression.

Here are the findings as to the side-effects of HRT:

- 85 per cent of patients suffered breast tenderness
- 72 per cent put on unwanted weight
- 39 per cent experienced mood swings
- 21 per cent experienced depression
- 17 per cent experienced a rise in blood pressure
- 6 per cent lost hair from their head
- 6 per cent had thrombosis.

It was interesting and enlightening to learn that the participating doctors were knowledgeable about, and even incorporated natural treatments for the menopause. More conventional treatments, such as Dixarit, a drug to alleviate hot flushes, appeared to be only 27 per cent effective. Advising their patients to reduce their consumption of caffeine, alcohol and cigarettes were nigh-on as effective for reducing flushes.

It was quite amazing to find that as many as 17 per cent of doctors were recommending a soy-rich diet, 18 per cent advised taking a phytoestrogen-rich diet, while only 8 per cent recommended vitamin supplements and referral for psychotherapy.

Since we carried out our first GP survey in 1994, it would seem that knowledge of complementary therapies for treating menopausal symptoms is increasing, perhaps not significantly, but at least the trend is moving in the right direction!

A major problem has been that the majority of studies performed to date have looked at the effects of HRT in women who themselves *chose* to take HRT and very often such women also *chose* to take more care of themselves. So it is not clear how much of the apparent improvement is actually due to HRT and how much to a better lifestyle characteristic of many HRT users. Only what are termed prospective randomised trials will tell us the answers and these are currently under way. In these trials the women are divided into two groups with characteristics in common, such as weight, smoking, and risk factors for heart disease, breast cancer and osteoporosis. Then those who will receive HRT are chosen randomly. These studies will need to contain many thousands of women and be conducted for 10 or more years before we have a complete answer.

Consequently, the existing information has to be assessed very carefully. In this chapter we will look at how HRT use should be viewed as a result of the trials and studies to date. The essential hormonal event at the time of the menopause is the decline in oestrogen level. This hormone influences the function and health of many tissues, including the uterus, breast, nervous system, blood vessels and bones. The decline in the level of oestrogen results in changes in these parts of the body and a variety of symptoms in the short term is added to the risk of osteoporosis and possibly heart disease in the long term. Giving replacement doses of oestrogen is highly effective in controlling hot flushes, nightsweats and vaginal dryness. However, unopposed oestrogen results in proliferation, and overgrowth of the lining of the womb and raises the risk of endometrial cancer. Therefore, women who take HRT who have not had a hysterectomy need to take progesterone on a cyclical basis, to induce shedding of the endometrial lining. This withdrawal bleed reduces the added risk of endometrial cancer developing.

Here are some important guiding principles concerning the use of HRT which should be at the forefront of any doctor's mind who is involved with this therapy.

GUIDING PRINCIPLES ON THE USE OF HRT

These are intended to help the patient (and doctor) to understand the appropriateness of HRT for her particular situation.

The two main indications for the administration of HRT are the control of menopausal symptoms and the treatment or prevention of postmenopausal osteoporosis

HRT is highly effective in the treatment of hot flushes, nightsweats and vaginal dryness and is quite effective in the treatment and prevention of osteoporosis in women who have been through the menopause. There may be other benefits from taking HRT over long term but at present this is uncertain. There is no basis for the routine prescribing of HRT to postmenopausal women.

Before HRT is prescribed,

- diagnosis of menopause or osteoporosis should be confirmed
- major contra-indications to HRT should be excluded (this includes examination of blood pressure, pelvic organs and breasts if there is a history of breast disease, and measurement of weight)
- risks and benefits of treatment should be discussed
- when appropriate, the therapies complementary and alternative to HRT should also be discussed.

The diagnosis of the menopause is usually straightforward

Typically, the picture is of cessation of menstruation or irregular menstruation together with the presence of hot flushes, nightsweats and, later on, vaginal dryness. However, other conditions can occasionally cause these symptoms (see below). Blood tests may occasionally be needed to confirm the diagnosis.

Not all menopausal symptoms are eased by HRT

There is no doubt that HRT has a high degree of success in treating hot flushes, nightsweats, the associated sleep disturbance and vaginal dryness. However, depression, anxiety, aches and pains, and changes in skin and hair are less dependably improved and mood changes may be worsened. It is inappropriate for any doctor or patient to expect these other symptoms to improve with HRT and their presence alone is not usually considered a good enough reason to prescribe it.

The diagnosis of osteoporosis depends upon measurement of bone mineral density

This specialised X-ray measures the density of bone at the hip and spine and compares the patients reading with the average for her age and that of the peak value achieved by younger women. Very low levels are termed osteoporosis and intermediate levels are termed osteopenia. Osteoporosis is a silent condition but can often be suspected because of the presence of several risk factors, for example, premature menopause, small frame, heavy smoking, immobility, poor diet, and others. At present there is no reliable, easy way to assess an individual's risk of osteoporosis without measuring her bone mineral density (BMD).

Not all women can be given HRT

There are a number of situations in which HRT cannot be prescribed and, should they develop during the course of treatment, then HRT will need to be stopped. These include:

- cancer of the breast, womb, ovary or other part of the genital tract, any other oestrogen-dependent tumour
- undiagnosed vaginal bleeding or endometriosis
- active thrombophlebitis
- deep vein thrombosis, known or suspected thromboembolic disorder (tendency to blood clotting)
- severe heart, liver or kidney disease and certain liver disorders
- pregnancy or lactation are also obvious contra-indications to HRT. High blood pressure is not necessarily a contra-indication but it will need to be controlled by diet or by medication. Any co-existent gynaecological disorder or breast abnormality will need to be assessed prior to commencing treatment.

There are many different forms of HRT

Tablets of varying type, patches, gels, and implant preparations all come with a choice of dose and can be provided in different combinations of oestrogen and progesterone. All are effective at controlling immediate symptoms and most are proven to have beneficial effects upon bone health. The wide choice means that there is considerable flexibility and gives the doctor many alternatives if one preparation is not well tolerated. Women with a uterus will need to take progesterone for 12 to 14 days per month to prevent endometrial overgrowth and cancer from developing. This applies also to those women receiving vaginal oestrogen preparations for more than three months.

HRT brings both short and long term benefits

In addition to the control of menopausal symptoms, HRT reduces the risk of osteoporotic fracture and *may* bring other benefits, including a reduction in the risk of heart disease and dementia, but this is by no means certain at present. Large detailed trials to answer these and other questions are under way in Europe and the United States. The results will not be available for several years.

HRT use can bring both short- and long-term health problems

Common initial side-effects include breast tenderness, aggravation of pre-existing breast disease, mood changes and, in those receiving cyclical progesterone, cyclical mood changes akin to premenstrual syndrome, headaches and irregular vaginal bleeding. These problems are, of course, similar to those experienced with the oral contraceptive pill. They may become tolerable, diminish with time or be controlled by a change in dose or preparation. The longer-term side-effects are more serious and include an increase in the risk of breast cancer and thrombosis.

To some degree the increased risks of breast cancer and thrombosis are predictable

The increase in breast cancer is between 10 and 20 per cent after 10 years' continuous use, with very little increase in the first five years. Furthermore five years after ceasing treatment, the risk returns to that of non-users. The increased risk of thrombosis (three in 10,000) may become apparent after just a few weeks of HRT. Occasionally, this may lead to a blood clot on the lung which in one to two per cent of cases can be fatal. The risk of thrombosis rises significantly with the higher-dose preparations, particularly if the woman is overweight, a smoker or has had a thrombosis in the past.

Some conditions call for additional attention on the part of the doctor

There are a number of situations where HRT is not prohibited but special care is required because there is either an increased risk of thrombosis developing or another condition may be aggravated by HRT. In the former category indicators are: being very overweight (Body Mass Index greater than 30) or being immobilised, especially if the woman is also a smoker, and following major trauma or surgery. In the latter category are a wide variety of conditions, including: uterine fibroids, mild chronic liver disease (blood tests to monitor liver function every eight to 12 weeks), gall stones, otosclerosis (hormone-dependent hearing loss), migraine, multiple sclerosis, epilepsy, diabetes, high blood pressure, kidney disease, the rare metabolic condition porphyria, and tetany.

For the control of menopausal symptoms, most women will need treatment for between one and five years

The majority of patients will be between 40 and mid-50s with younger patients typically having more severe symptoms that often require a higher dose of HRT and for longer. Stopping treatment after a maximum of five years will minimise the increase in the risk of breast cancer and thrombosis and by this time many symptoms will have lessened. Younger patients with a premature menopause (before the age of 45) may well need or wish to take it for longer. However, as a rule it would seem inappropriate to continue HRT past the age of 55 unless a woman is known to have or is at high risk of developing osteoporosis, and even then, there now exist alternative approaches, as you will see in Chapter 9.

The treatment of established osteoporosis and its prevention takes between five and 10 years

The majority of such patients will be elderly and five years is probably the minimum period to achieve a reasonable effect. Going beyond 10 years may either not be necessary or may add to the risk of breast cancer and thrombosis with little additional benefit in terms of bone protection.

The benefits of HRT can be found elsewhere

There are alternatives to HRT of a pharmaceutical and non-pharmaceutical nature. Hot flushes can be helped by a low dose of the drug Clonidine, by relaxation techniques and dietary change, including the consuming of certain foods or preparations containing phytoestrogens which in part perform some of the functions of HRT (see Chapter 8). Osteoporosis can be treated by other drugs, calcium with additional vitamin D for the elderly, and helped by regular exercise. Furthermore, regular exercise and a healthy diet will almost certainly protect against both osteoporosis and heart disease to at least the same extent as HRT and bring with it many additional benefits, see Chapter 9. If a doctor is prescribing HRT for its long-term preventative benefits, then he or she should also be advising about other ways to minimise the development of both osteoporosis and heart disease.

Certain situations call for the immediate cessation of HRT

This is needed if there is:

- a thrombosis, a blood clot in any part of the body – leg, lung, brain or heart, or if there is an injury which is likely to result in a thrombosis
- severe migraine headaches developing for the first time or any other frequent or severe headaches, especially if they are associated with visual disturbance or the development of symptoms such as numbness or tingling in a part of the body
- the development of jaundice, high blood pressure or pregnancy are all reasons to stop HRT without delay
- HRT should also be stopped six weeks before any operation or if there is prolonged immobilisation.

Abrupt cessation of HRT can cause a marked return in symptoms

Research shows that women who come off HRT suddenly often experience severe hot flushing. The return of hot flushes and nightsweats when HRT is stopped abruptly is not 'proof' of oestrogen deficiency but merely testimony to the intolerance of many women's bodies to sudden and substantial hormonal change. Gradually reducing the dose may produce fewer symptoms and may need to be done for many women coming off HRT in their early to mid-fifties. Some of these women may return to HRT a decade or two later for the treatment/prevention of their osteoporosis.

The duration of HRT treatment often cannot be decided until after an initial test phase

Only after several months of trying HRT can the full balance between risks and benefits for the individual be assessed, especially if it has been necessary to adjust the dose or type of HRT to control initial, adverse symptoms. This means that each woman should be advised when commencing treatment that she is not necessarily committing herself to long-term treatment but actually undertaking a therapeutic trial. At the end of the first few months or year of treatment there can then be a more detailed assessment of the appropriateness of continuing with HRT in the medium to long term.

ASSESSING THE APPROPRIATENESS OF HRT

Having absorbed these guiding principles we can now make some kind of planned approach to assessing the appropriateness of HRT for an individual woman. A lot of the following factors will need to be considered in the logical sequence presented here. Each case should be considered as a therapeutic trial unique to that individual.

Step 1 – Initial assessment

Blood tests to diagnose the menopause
The tests at the GP's disposal, to confirm a diagnosis of 'menopausal' are as follows:

- **FSH** and **LH** These are tests of pituitary function and will be elevated as the pituitary gland works hard to try to stimulate the failing ovary. In perimenopausal women these levels rise before the oestrogen level falls
- **Oestradiol** This is the main type of oestrogen in the body and levels will fall at the time of the menopause. A low normal level, in conjunction with elevations of FSH/LH, are found in perimenopausal women
- **Other tests** Most commonly these will include blood tests of thyroid function and anaemia, especially if some other health problem is also suspected. Other tests will rarely be needed.

Should the woman be given an initial trial of HRT?
This should be considered if there are symptoms of hot flushes, nightsweats or vaginal dryness. These are archetypal symptoms of

oestrogen withdrawal. Other symptoms such as depression, low libido and muscular aches and pains have many other causes and by themselves are not a good guide as to the suitability of HRT. Or if there is a likelihood of developing osteoporosis, especially if combined with an early menopause. It should also be considered if there are no major contra-indications to HRT or if there is a relative contra-indication to HRT but she is willing to accept the associated increased risks.

An initial trial could also be given if the individual is psychologically prepared to take HRT. This means that she has not been scared off by stories that she has heard or read and is willing to accept the use of a short-term physiological replacement. Importantly, there should be no pressure for her to agree to take it on a long-term basis until she has seen how she gets on with it in the short term.

The contra-indications listed below are taken from standard texts, including the prescribing handbook, the Monthly Index of Medical Specialities (MIMS) which sits at the elbow of most consulting doctors, and from the relevant reference texts.

Major contra-indications to HRT
Some women should not even consider trying HRT. This is because they have a pre-existing condition that is likely to be worsened by HRT or they have a history of marked intolerance of oestrogen preparations.

- **Pre-existing breast cancer** The growth of breast cancer is usually hormone-dependent, especially in young women and HRT would conflict with treatment for the cancer, especially with the oestrogen-modulating drug Tamoxifen
- **Pre-existing uterine, ovarian, or cervical cancer** Again, these are hormone-dependent cancers and HRT should not be given
- **Undiagnosed vaginal bleeding** This could be due to cancer of the genital tract. Heavy or erratic bleeding or bleeding after intercourse should arouse suspicion
- **Endometriosis** When the endometrial lining has extended outside the womb there is usually considerable abdominal pain with menstruation and, typically, a day before the onset of bleeding. Abdominal pain and swelling are likely to worsen with HRT.
- **Previous thrombosis when taking oestrogen** Oestrogen causes an increase in blood-clotting factors which, in a few individuals, will lead to a blood clot developing in a vein, a venous thrombosis, which will cause a swollen and usually painful leg. However, sometimes this process is silent until a clot breaks off and travels to the lung, causing a pulmonary embolus. If large, this may occasionally be

fatal. Smaller clots will usually cause chest pain, shortness of breath and a cough, often resulting in blood-stained sputum. Multiple small pulmonary emboli, if unrecognised, can damage the lung and heart. The risk of thrombosis rises with increasing age, obesity, smoking, immobility, recent trauma or surgery, and any of several otherwise silent blood conditions that predispose to blood clotting. These may only be suspected because of a previous personal history of thrombosis, especially in association with the oral contraceptive pill or HRT or because a first degree relative has suffered a thrombosis spontaneously or when taking an oestrogen preparation. Rarely such individuals may have experienced a stroke or stroke-like episode when on the oral contraceptive pill. Sophisticated and expensive blood tests exist to detect the different forms of thrombophilia, as these blood conditions are known. However, they are not widely available, which is a situation that will have to change in the future.

- *Active thrombosis or embolism* For the same reasons
- *Severe migraine or visual disturbance when taking the oral contraceptive pill* These symptoms could mean an impending stroke linked to increased risk of thrombosis when taking the pill
- *Severe heart, kidney or liver disease* HRT can aggravate the fluid retention that occurs with these conditions
- *Some liver diseases* These may alter the metabolism of oestrogen
- *Pregnancy or lactation* Not all older women have ceased menstruating because of the menopause. It is prudent to enquire whether they might be pregnant!
- *Likely to have an operation within the next six weeks* An operation increases the risk of thrombosis and whenever possible HRT should not be taken during this time.

Relative contra-indications to HRT
These conditions will usually have been previously diagnosed in the individual because of some prior episode of ill health. They include:

- *Uterine fibroids* which could cause heavier bleeding as a result of HRT use
- *Mild chronic liver disease* further monitoring of liver function tests will be needed every eight to 12 weeks
- *Gall stones*
- *Porphyria* a rare metabolic condition that alters liver metabolism
- *Otosclerosis* deafness in pregnancy or in association with the oral contraceptive pill
- *Hypertension* rarely, this may be made worse by HRT

- **Migraine** which again may be made worse by HRT
- **Epilepsy** might be made worse by HRT and some anti-epileptic drugs will increase the required HRT dose
- **Multiple sclerosis** may very rarely be worsened by HRT
- **Diabetes** there may be minor changes in blood sugar control following treatment with HRT
- **Renal impairment** HRT might aggravate fluid retention
- **Premenstrual syndrome** either currently or in the past may mean that the woman will be prone to cyclical mood changes when taking HRT. This is quite variable and not easily predictable, but it is thought that one third of women who try HRT can expect to experience premenstrual symptoms
- **Breast cysts or pain** either may worsen with HRT. All sufferers should be examined before commencing treatment and, if the diagnosis is in doubt, be sent for mammography
- **A strong family history of breast cancer** The increased risk of breast cancer developing following the use of HRT is small, especially when it is only taken for a short period of time, but not insignificant. In women with a strong family history of this cancer, careful and sympathetic discussion is often required, and alternative approaches may well be preferred.

Most of these points can be quickly assessed by your own family doctor. The most tricky one is when there is a personal or family history of thrombosis as at present there are no clear guidelines as to how to assess the risk in individual cases.

Step 2 – The choice of HRT

There are a wide variety of HRT preparations to consider and choices to be made, including:

- The route of administration
- Bleed or no-bleed systems
- The dose
- Lifestyle advice for women on HRT.

Route of administration
This is often a matter for personal preference:

- **Tablets** are the commonest form

- **Patches** have the advantage of by-passing the liver and this may reduce some of the side-effects, although some women are allergic to the patches
- **Gels and creams** applied to the skin are not always suitable in hot climates
- **Implants** provide HRT for approximately six months, but if side-effects occur they will need to be surgically removed. A blood test to measure the level of oestrogen is necessary before subsequent implants are given to prevent excessive administration of the hormone.

Bleed or no-bleed systems

For those with a uterus the oestrogen must be combined with progesterone in some form to prevent overgrowth of the uterine lining which could lead to cancer. The different preparations allow further choice between monthly bleed, three-monthly bleed and no-bleed preparations suitable for older women who have gone for a year without a period.

The dose

Often there is not a lot of choice but there is usually some. This is important as:

- Oestrogen requirements vary from person to person
- Younger people with more severe symptoms generally need a higher dose of HRT
- Some of the side-effects are related to the dose of HRT
- Dietary and other factors can alter the required dose of HRT
- Lower doses carry less risk of thrombosis and can still be very effective.

Once the initial choice has been made and the trial begins, there should usually be a follow up appointment in approximately six to eight weeks to assess progress and suitability.

Lifestyle advice for women on HRT

This should ideally be given to all women receiving HRT.

- **Watch your weight** Being overweight adds to the risk of thrombosis as well as high blood pressure
- **Do not drink alcohol excessively** i.e., more than 10 units per week (1 glass of wine = 1 unit). High intakes of alcohol will temporarily raise the level of oestrogen threefold. Erratic swings in the level of oestrogen may reduce the effectiveness of HRT in controlling

symptoms. Furthermore, high intakes of alcohol add considerably to the risk of breast cancer

- **Do not smoke** Smoking increases the risk of thrombosis and osteoporosis as well as heart disease
- **Eat a healthy diet** Include lots of vegetables, fruit and calcium-rich foods, particularly if you have osteoporosis
- **Do not drink coffee excessively** This will aggravate hot flushes
- **Exercise regularly** 30 minutes of weight-bearing exercise, e.g., brisk walking for 20 minutes five days a week is now the minimum recommended for the prevention of osteoporosis
- *Women on HRT should also note that: diarrhoea or antibiotics may temporarily lower the level of oestrogen and prompt a return of symptoms*
- *They should use contraception if appropriate*
- *They should stop taking HRT six weeks before any planned operation*
- *They should stop taking HRT and report immediately to their doctor if one of the major contra-indications develops*
- *They should avoid reading extremist articles for or against HRT if they want a peaceful life!*

Step 3 – The first follow-up

The purpose of this assessment at six to eight weeks is to assess the effectiveness of the initial response to HRT in controlling menopausal symptoms. If this is inadequate, a higher dose or change in type may need to be prescribed. It is also necessary to assess the initial side-effects of HRT which include the exacerbation of pre-existing gynaecological conditions (this will typically cause pain or, rarely, heavy bleeding). Other side-effects, which can be quite severe in some individuals, include:

- breast tenderness or enlargement
- mood changes
- nausea
- slight weight gain
- mild headache – possibly due to high blood pressure
- breakthrough bleeding
- dizziness, erythema of the face or hands
- increased facial pigmentation
- alterations in blood sugar tolerance.

These may settle in time or respond to a change in dose or type of the HRT.

The more serious side-effects include; venous thrombosis, most commonly in the leg and, occasionally, elsewhere. The risk of this developing is very small. Should this happen it will call for an immediate cessation in treatment and usually no attempt to retry further HRT preparations without expert assessment. Blood pressure which will rise in about one per cent of patients to a level that means that the HRT may have to be stopped. These women may have experienced a similar problem with the oral contraceptive pill. They should not pass undetected. In those for whom it is perceived that HRT is essential, then control of the blood pressure through diet and drugs will be necessary but for some it may be difficult to continue on HRT.

Those with relative contra-indications to HRT will need further monitoring (e.g., liver function tests, jaundice tests, blood glucose level monitoring). Lifestyle changes (e.g., cessation of smoking, weight reduction, ensuring good dietary intake of calcium and other important nutrients, or compliance with calcium supplementation) will need to be checked. Any further questions about HRT will need to be answered as this will help to maintain compliance with the treatment. At this first follow-up it may be a good idea to discuss further how long the woman wants to, or will need to take it for.

The initial duration of HRT will need to be determined. Typically, this will be for several months to years for those who need control of menopausal symptoms, and for five to 10 years for those who have or are at risk of osteoporosis, unless an alternative method is employed (see Chapter 9).

66 Margaret's Story 99

Margaret, a 51-year-old nursery teacher from Hertfordshire, came to the WNAS with menopausal symptoms, and also suffered with irritable bowel syndrome (IBS).

'About four years ago my GP recommended HRT patches for my menopausal symptoms. I ballooned within six to eight months from 10 1/2 stone to 14 stone. My breathing deteriorated and I am sure it was around this time that I started to experience IBS. After a long debate with my doctor I stopped using HRT and lost 1 1/2 stone within weeks! This was great, but the dreadful hot *flushes came back. A friend told me to take supplements which had been use-ful to her, and at that time I read about the work of the WNAS in the Mail on Sunday You Magazine, so I decided to get in touch with them.*

I had tried so many things to control my IBS, and in the end I was told to live with the condition which was extremely disheartening. My main concern was the abdominal bloating, excessive wind and severe constipation which was causing great embarrassment. When the constipation was really severe, it triggered an outbreak of piles and my doctor repeatedly recommended eat-ing a high-fibre diet with plenty of bran and wholewheat. I followed his advice, but the diet seemed to worsen my symptoms and leave me doubled up with pain.

I wrote to the WNAS briefly explaining my problems and they sent details of their organisation and a very comprehensive Menopause Questionnaire and seven-day diet diary for me to complete. I diligently filled in the forms and returned them straight away. A consultation with the nutritionist was arranged for the following week. The consultation was held over the tele-phone, lasting approximately 40 minutes, and it was recommended that I should exclude wheat, oats, barley and rye from my diet. It seemed a little confusing – the WNAS recommended a diet avoiding all wheat and bran, while the doctor was telling me to eat more of it! Maryon explained very clear-ly that these grains can in fact aggravate IBS symptoms and cause all the symptoms that I was experiencing. It was also recommended that I increase my intake of phytoestrogens which would help to regulate my own body's nat-ural oestrogen levels. I had to take nutritional supplements to control the symptoms which really helped the hot flushes and nightsweats.

I had a follow-up consultation after two months of rigorously following the programme. Following the IBS dietary programme was more difficult than I imagined, but my weight was slowing going down (7lbs in the first two months) and my bloating was definitely under control. Cutting out all dairy products, wheat, oats, barley and rye changed my entire approach to eating, but the immense benefits made me persevere.

Another two months into the programme and I was like a new woman! My husband had noticed a difference, especially my weight loss. When I enrolled on the programme my weight was 13st 4lb and after four months I had lost more than two stone! My severe to moderate menopausal symptoms were previously problematic every day. On the WNAS programme they reduced to occasional symptoms scoring 'mild to none'.

I cannot believe I put up with the pain and embarrassment of my IBS for so many years. Looking back, it seems so obvious that I was being "fobbed off" by the medical profession, and only wish I had approached the WNAS sooner. Enrolling on the programme was the best thing I have ever done. I am marvelling at how everything settled down so quickly.'

Step 4 – Longer-term monitoring of women on HRT

By this stage the majority of women who have remained on HRT are satisfied with their HRT preparation and will only need occasional monitoring, which should include:

- *Blood pressure measurement* approximately once a year
- *Weighing* yearly or more frequently if overweight, together with encouragement to lose weight
- *Breast examination and mammography* every three years, although those women with breast cysts or pre-existing breast disease will need more frequent examinations. In approximately one third of women, HRT will make the breast appear more dense on mammography. This feature is associated with a doubling of the risk of breast cancer, although the overall risk is still small
- *Cervical smears* every three years but more frequently in those with abnormal smears
- *Bone mineral density examinations* for most of those who are being treated for established osteoporosis and in some who are taking HRT for its prevention, particularly if they have many predisposing factors or a chronic condition that adds significantly to the risk. The interval for repeat BMD varies between one and five years. A poor response may mean an increase in the dose of HRT, the addition of supplemental calcium, encouragement to do more exercise or a review of the possible cause(s) of the patient's osteoporosis
- *Other tests* that may be necessary if there is also a relative contraindication, e.g., liver or kidney disease
- *Review of treatment in the light of new research* is important as there are still many unanswered questions about the longer-term use of HRT which will probably be addressed by the results of trials currently in progress. This may well cause a change in the type, dose or duration of HRT administration for some women.

Step 5 – Coming off HRT

Eventually, most women will need to stop HRT; those taking it for the control of menopausal symptoms may not wish or need to take it for more than a few years and it would seem reasonable not to continue it past the age of 55, unless there is a genuine need to protect them from osteoporosis. Older women with established osteoporosis or who are in need of active prevention are advised to take it for between five and 10 years. However, research is now showing that there are scientifically based non-drug preparations, rich in isoflavones, that help successfully to regenerate bone tissue. The long-term studies, over 20 years, are now showing that HRT only produces a three per cent greater bone mass than found in those women not taking HRT. We know that exercise, diets rich in calcium, fish oils and phytoestrogens, plus isoflavone-rich supplements all help to regenerate lost bone significantly. It is therefore fair to say that osteoporosis can be prevented, and even treated in the early stages quite successfully without having to resort to HRT.

Additionally, there will be few who will need to stop their HRT as a matter of urgency because of the development of a major contra-indication. This is more likely to happen in the elderly on long-term treatment than in younger women. The main reasons for stopping HRT are:

- *Development of an absolute contra-indication* as detailed above. The most likely are breast or genital tract cancer, vaginal bleeding of uncertain origin, a thrombosis or active thrombophlebitis, severe migraine with visual or other localised neurological features, severe heart, liver or kidney disease, or pregnancy. These events should all be rare. However, with long-term administration in older people, there is an increasing likelihood of some of these situations occurring. In all of these situations the withdrawal of HRT will have to be immediate and the woman may well experience hot flushes and nightsweats as part of the acute withdrawal reaction.

- *Planned withdrawal due to* increasing age and unwillingness to continue with HRT; adequate response in the treatment of osteoporosis; inadequate response in the treatment of osteoporosis with necessary replacement by other treatments, especially calcium, phytoestrogen-rich supplements, bisphosphonates and exercise.

Other planned withdrawal circumstances are: a forthcoming planned operation, in which case HRT should be withdrawn six weeks before the date of the operation. It could then be reintroduced once the woman is fully mobile, approximately two to four weeks after the operation. If there is a prolonged period of immobility, e.g., because of illness or following a fracture, with increased risk of thrombosis, then planned temporary withdrawal of HRT will be appropriate. Withdrawal will also be appropriate if a relative contra-indication develops, e.g., mild liver disease or severe or worsening heart failure; if there are persistent and unacceptable side-effects (but this should be rare at this stage); and finally, if there is a supervening condition, e.g., terminal illness or dementia.

« Nicola's Story »

Nicola is a 46-year-old mother of two and part-time conference organ-iser who approached the WNAS in September 1997.

'At the age of 44 I began experiencing hot flushes and nightsweats. I felt depressed so my doctor prescribed antidepressants and in addition I felt bloated and constipated. I also had constant aches and pains. A blood test confirmed an early menopause. I tried HRT but within days was experiencing panic attacks and depression, and feeling totally out of control and suicidal. Within one week I had stopped the HRT and took several weeks to regain my composure. After coming off the HRT I experienced hot and cold flushes, nightsweats, headaches, constipation, general aches and pains and persistent depression.

At my initial consultation, dietary modifications were made and it was rec-ommended that I take nutritional supplements. The WNAS put me on a phy-toestrogen-rich diet of soy milk, tofu, alfalfa and other phyto-rich foods. I was a little apprehensive, but was prepared to try anything to relieve my symptoms.

One month later at my follow-up consultation, I was able to report increased energy and a more positive outlook on life. My symptoms were diminishing by the week. I travel quite frequently with my job, but managed to stick to the recommendations by taking with me a good supply of soy milk and rice cakes!

Four months down the line I continued to improve, feeling mentally more alert, more in control and the constipation was a thing of the past. A bonus of following the WNAS programme was weight loss of more than a stone. My family and colleagues have also noticed a more rational person in their midst!'

How to withdraw from HRT

In those taking cyclical progesterone, HRT can be stopped at the end of the progesterone phase. Those just taking oestrogen can stop at any time, but research shows that it is best done gradually. Those who develop an absolute contra-indication will need to stop regardless of where they are in the hormonal cycle. However younger women, those on higher doses and those who were severely troubled by hot flushes and nightsweats, may well experience acute withdrawal symptoms, with sudden severe hot flushes, possibly accompanied by sleep distur-bance and mood changes. In these circumstances phased withdrawal over two or three months may be necessary. If this is difficult to achieve in those using oral preparations, it may be helpful to change to low-dose patch or gel systems. We successfully wean our patients off HRT over a month or two by using ever-decreasing doses whilst getting them established on the WNAS Menopause Programme.

Altering the dose of HRT

Most forms of HRT are presented either with no choice of dose or a choice between two strengths. As there is considerable variation in sensitivity to, and tolerance of, both oestrogen and progesterone, there often needs to be some adjustment. Unlike thyroid hormone replacement therapy, actual levels of oestrogen are rarely measured and the woman's testimony of her response to treatment is usually taken as a guide to dosage adequacy.

There are certain circumstances when it is likely that the dose of HRT will need to be altered.

Increasing the dose of HRT

Conventional doctors are likely to suggest an increase in the dosage in the following circumstances:

- Hot flushes, nightsweats, vaginal dryness and other menopause-related symptoms are inadequately controlled by the existing HRT dose. Other conditions, including an overactive thyroid or a fever, can also point to apparent HRT failure. We at the WNAS would suggest incorporating phytoestrogens into the diet, and a whole host of other scientifically based non-drug measures that help to control the short-term symptoms of the menopause, as you will see from the recommendations in Parts Three and Four of this book
- If bone mineral density fails to improve adequately in those with osteoporosis (a two per cent response per year can be expected during treatment with HRT). Again, other unrelated conditions should be considered. In addition, the WNAS would make a number of recommendations which have been shown to increase bone density considerably (see page 134 for further details)
- If the woman is also taking a drug which accelerates the breakdown of oestrogens in the liver, e.g., anti-epileptic drugs, certain antibiotics used in the treatment of tuberculosis, and others. Short courses of antibiotics, e.g., amoxycillin for one week in premenopausal women can certainly lower oestrogen levels temporarily. Most courses of antibiotics do not necessitate a change in HRT dose although they might slightly alter the level of hormone-related symptoms.

Those on long-term antibiotics may need further advice and assessment, including measurement of relevant hormone levels.

Decreasing the dose of HRT

This may need to be done when:

- There are troublesome oestrogen-related side-effects, especially breast tenderness and nausea. This is most likely when first commencing HRT and may settle with time. A lower dose or preparation may be needed, or switching to a patch preparation may be an option
- Alcohol consumption is chronically high, as this retards the clearance of HRT by the liver and may contribute to increased levels of oestrogen
- Liver disease is present which will again slow down the clearance of HRT from the body
- The need for the higher doses of HRT that women under the age of fifty sometimes require declines with increasing age.

Women who are receiving oestrogen implants still have a high level of oestrogen prior to receiving their next implant, so oestrogen levels in the patient's blood should be routinely checked and the next implant should only be given if the level has fallen to the required value. Repeatedly administering oestrogen implants when the level of oestrogen is already adequate or high will result in reduced therapeutic benefit and increasing side-effects, or a condition called tachyphylaxis which will then need to be followed by a prolonged phase of often troublesome withdrawal. I had one patient who had 22 implants removed from her abdomen after constantly complaining of feeling unwell. Her oestrogen levels were measured at around 8000 which dramatically exceeds the normal range of around 300.

In our long experience in treating women experiencing symptoms of the menopause, we have found that the vast majority manage to overcome their symptoms extremely well, and in a relatively short space of time, without using HRT. As well as controlling the symptoms of the menopause, our alternative approach alleviates the worry about the potential long-term side-effects of HRT. In Parts Three and Four you will find all the components of the successful WNAS Menopause Programme outlined.

6
NUTRITION AND HEALTH

So far, we have been looking at the mechanics of the menopause and how some of the symptoms in some women could be helped by oestrogen replacement. But in doing so, we discovered that some of the symptoms are not particularly related to a fall in oestrogen levels, and thus there must be some other underlying cause.

What we haven't inspected closely is our diet and lifestyle and the relationship they have to our health and well-being, or lack of it. Our 21st-century diet is very different from that of our ancestors.

When we examine our early ancestors' diet, we begin to realise that it is not 'natural' to eat meat protein, for instance, in the quantity that many of us do today. Evidence shows that approximately three million years ago diet consisted largely of hard seeds, plant fibre, some roots and stems – i.e., a diet high in vegetable matter.

Animals today are bred to be fat. Modern meat contains considerably more fat than the wild meat our ancestors ate. Our ancestors' meat also contained more of the good polyunsaturated fats than today's meat, which is high in potentially harmful saturated fats. The ancient diet was also richer in vitamins and minerals, largely composed of fresh, raw foods.

Lifestyle is different too, for as recently as the 1930s, approximately four 'proper' meals were consumed each day, with only one or two in-between-meal snacks, whereas now we consume an average of one or two proper meals a day, with approximately four or five in-between-meal snacks. Convenience food and pre-prepared meals are often served instead of wholesome home cooking, largely because time is at a premium.

We no longer have the extended family to fall back on and very often women have to be the wage-earner now, as well as *Hausfrau* and mother.

We exercise far less as well. In the age of the motor car, many of us have forgotten what our legs were designed for. We drive from one place to another, do more sitting down than is good for us and allow our metabolic rate to rest!

The net result is that we are suffering far more from conditions that were not so common in the past. Heart disease, cancer, diabetes and osteoporosis are just a few of the disorders that are on the increase. So too are symptoms like irritable bowel syndrome, including constipation, diarrhoea with a painful and windy, bloated abdomen, migraine headaches, nervous tension, irritability, insomnia, feelings of aggression and fatigue.

THE MIDLIFE SURVEY

In August 1999 we conducted a survey of women at midlife in order to assess their health prospects. We analysed a thousand of them. 51 per cent were still menstruating, and 57 per cent said they wouldn't contemplate taking Hormone Replacement Therapy during their menopause.

- A staggering 73 per cent of the women included in the sample admitted not feeling as healthy as they used to, with only 27 per cent doing adequate exercise.

- 15 per cent of the sample were smokers, with 68 per cent smoking more than 10 cigarettes per day. Interestingly, the smokers were more concerned about the prospects of contracting cancer than they were about heart disease, and they were hardly concerned at all about osteoporosis.

- On a more positive note, 93 per cent of the women said they were willing to modify their diet, 92 per cent were willing to increase their exercise, and 89 per cent were willing to incorporate relaxation into their timetable.

Our conclusion in general, bearing in mind that some 83 per cent had never heard of phytoestrogens, was that the underlying cause for their decreased well-being was a lack of education. In our experience, once this is remedied, the women themselves soon greatly improve their long-term health prospects.

Let's just take a quick look at some of the major problems and how they are influenced by our diet and lifestyle.

THE PRICE OF ILLNESS

Heart disease

Cardiovascular disease is still the biggest killer in developed countries and undoubtedly the commonest preventable cause of early death in young to middle-aged men and women. Approximately 300,000 people die each year in the UK from heart attacks and strokes. There has been little improvement, as yet, in these figures, although the USA and Finland have begun to achieve a substantial fall in their incidence of heart disease. Smoking, lack of exercise, obesity, high blood pressure and high blood cholesterol are all well-documented risk factors and these last three are all influenced by diet.

Cancer

Cancer, too, it appears, is on the increase. There seem to be three main factors for this. The first is age. With a few exceptions, the incidence of most cancers rises steeply with age from about the age of 40. In the past, many people did not live long enough to be at risk of developing cancer. Second, it is highly likely that there has been a true increase in the rate of cancer this century, regardless of age, and that this reflects the increased use of chemicals in the environment. Many industrial chemicals, pesticides and even drugs linger in the environment for years.

Finally, the type of food we eat also influences cancer risk. Consumption of smoked and pickled foods is associated with an increase in some cancers, especially of the stomach and oesophagus, while a high intake of fresh fruit and vegetables may well protect against many types of cancer. These protective foods are rich in vitamins C, E and carotene – vegetable vitamin A – which help to limit the damage to tissues by cancer-inducing chemicals.

Psychiatric Illnesses

'Mental' illnesses are also on the increase and this too may be influenced by our diet, consumption of alcohol, medical and illicit drugs. Obviously, social factors, education and life-skills are also all-important in helping us to cope with times of stress or ill-health. The stresses and strains of 21st-century living have not made it easy for some of us to cope and for many women, working and raising a family and coping with aged relatives proves to be particularly stressful.

Allergies

Allergic problems have also become much more common in the last 40 years. The reasons for this are not clear but they include family or genetic factors, chemicals in the environment, dietary habits and the pattern of feeding in childhood.

MENOPAUSAL SYMPTOMS, DIET AND LIFESTYLE

What, I hear you ask, has this pessimistic view of the state of our health got to do with the menopause? Quite simply, it appears that the development of symptoms at the time of the menopause may very well be influenced by the same factors: diet, exercise or the lack of it and possibly environmental chemicals. It is possible that these diverse conditions have common causative and aggravating factors.

In 1990 the Women's Nutritional Advisory Service completed a national survey of 274 women in the UK in conjunction with a national newspaper. We found that 86.8 per cent of them suffered in varying degrees with symptoms at the time of the menopause. This figure concurs with other reported surveys. Over two-thirds of the women in our sample suffered with hot flushes or nightsweats. Fatigue was the next most commonly complained-about problem, followed by sexual problems and weight-gain. These are not all oestrogen-withdrawal symptoms, but can all be influenced by diet, as you will see.

Our bodies were not built to cope with refined and processed foods, very often empty of nutrients. We have had to live with pesticides and insecticides being sprayed on our crops, with growth hormones and antibiotics pumped into animals, and with environmental pollution and acid rain as the finishing touches. Many of us overeat and under-exercise and women nowadays tend to lead far more stressful existences. So we can't honestly expect our 'machines' to go on indefinitely without breaking down when we don't treat them with respect. We generally treat our cars better than we do our bodies – you wouldn't dream of putting the wrong fuel in your petrol tank, would you?

In order to look at diet more closely we need to examine how our habits have changed. As little as 100 years ago, meat, animal fat and sugar formed a much smaller part of our diet than today. The consumption of cereal fibres has also dropped considerably. These are important factors in relation to the menopause, as we shall see.

These days, in order to eat a 'normal, healthy diet' we have to pay far more attention to the foods and drinks we choose. If you concentrate on avoiding the nutrient-deficient and contaminated foods we have listed, you will be making changes for the better in your diet – changes which will not only help your menopause symptoms, but will help you feel healthier all round. There is less you can do to combat the unhealthy effects of our polluted environment, but there are some suggestions in the pages that follow.

- We have increased our consumption of sugar. The UK has become one of the world's largest chocolate and sweet-eaters, with the average person consuming some 188 lb or 85 kilos each per year. We currently spend over £3.2 billion per year on chocolate alone.
- Our diet is particularly high in saturated fats (animal fats). It is thought that this has much to do with our also having a high incidence of heart disease and breast cancer.
- We eat far too much salt – 10 to 20 times more than our bodies really require each day. Salt can contribute to high blood pressure and increase the risk of osteoporosis. Reduce the amount of salt used in cooking and at the table. Avoid salted foods such as salted nuts, kippers and bacon. Salt causes fluid retention and induces calcium loss from the urine. LoSalt is low-sodium, potassium-rich and makes a good substitute without the inherent problems associated with table salt. LoSalt is widely available from both supermarkets and health-food shops.
- We often drink far too much coffee and tea which can impede the absorption of essential nutrients and aggravate hot flushes, symptoms of irritability, nervous tension, insomnia and headaches. On average we consume four mugs of tea and two mugs of coffee each day, which delivers approximately 660 mg of caffeine into our system each day. Anything over 250 each day can give symptoms of caffeine excess, and that's in a healthy individual who has no existing symptoms. Count the number of teas and coffees you have had so far today; you may be consuming even more than average.
- We consume volumes of foods with a high level of phosphorus, which again impedes the absorption of good nutrients and interferes with calcium absorption by bone tissue. Examples of these foods are soft drinks of low or normal calorie types, processed foods, canned, packaged, prepacked convenience foods and ready-made sauces.
- Alcohol consumption has almost doubled in the UK since the end of the Second World War. Alcohol not only knocks most nutrients sideways, it also can bring on the hot flushes.

- Unbelievable as it may seem, we actually eat less food than we did 30 years ago and more. It seems that today's women actually expend less energy than those of a generation or two ago and this has resulted in a 10–15 per cent reduction in food intake. This means that our intake of essential nutrients has also fallen, particularly if we eat refined or convenience foods.
- Many of the foods available contain chemical additives in the form of flavour enhancers, colouring and preservatives. While some of these are not harmful, some of them are and our bodies are certainly not designed to cope with them.
- Our water contains certain pollutants which are thought to be a risk to public health.
- Our meat has become contaminated with antibiotics and growth hormones, so much so that vegetarians now have an easier menopause than meat-eaters.
- Nitrate fertilisers have been used to obtain fast-growing and abundant crops. It is now recognised that nitrates are harmful and can produce cancer, at least in animals.
- Almost all our fresh fruit, cereals and vegetables are sprayed with pesticides at least once. In addition, milk and meat may retain the pesticides from feed given to livestock.

Antibiotics

Because antibiotics are being so widely used on animals, the conditions that would normally be treated by antibiotics are becoming resistant to them. Apart from being used as a medicine for individual sick animals, they are given to whole herds as a preventive measure and they are again used for growth promotion.

My advice is to try to use organic or additive-free meat where possible – meat which has not been subjected to drugs, growth promoters or contaminated foods. Organic and additive-free meat is becoming more widely available. Certainly local farms and even supermarkets often keep stocks. If you can find 'clean' meat, it can be included in your diet approximately three times a week. An alternative is to limit your meat intake to moderate quantities of good-quality, lean meat or to become a vegetarian. It's the fat in the meat that will carry much of the pollutants, so avoid it – and also eat more fish. When eating chicken, don't eat the skin and don't make the gravy from the fatty part of the juices: pour it off first.

Genetic engineering

When soy is modified to make it resistant to an all-purpose weedkiller herbicide, there is a risk that the plant could contain higher levels of residues which, in turn, could worsen allergies in some and cause skin problems in others. Whilst the Monsanto Roundup soy bean has been declared safe to eat by American and European regulatory bodies, concerned nutritionists argue that food gene technology is still so new that the long-term risks are not quantifiable. The WNAS advise patients to avoid genetically modified soy products and to buy either organic soy or products that have a label stating that they do not use genetically engineered ingredients.

The Women's Nutritional Advisory Service carried out a survey to determine which manufacturers used genetically modified (GM) foods and ingredients and which didn't. Because the GMO scene is rapidly changing, and many food retailers were in the transitional stages of phasing out their GM stocks whilst trying to source new supplies, we felt it appropriate not to publish the results of the survey. Within one year of conducting the survey, we have seen an encouraging trend in the response to genetic engineering from the major food manufacturers and retailers. The general consensus now is that the main food manufacturers and supermarkets have either withdrawn all genetically engineered foods or they are in the transitional stages of removing them.

Fat consumption

Britain has the honour of having the highest incidence of heart disease in the world. This was not so in the past, when other countries such as Finland and Australia were way ahead.

It seems that the saturated fats increase the level of cholesterol which leaves the bloodstream and settles down in the arteries, resulting in a gradual blockage of those supplying the heart, brain and other organs. This leads to heart attacks, strokes and poor circulation. It is worth noting that smoking accelerates the process.

By 1966 the Australian and US rate of heart disease began to decline, but that was not so for the UK, whose casualties were on the increase. In other countries, such as Finland, for example, which was previously 'top of the coronary pops', a national nutritional education campaign was undertaken. The result is that today it is a much healthier nation with a far lower incidence of heart disease than many other countries.

The sweet facts

Over the past 100 years there has been a 25-fold increase in world sugar production. This is a real change from the days when sugar was an expensive luxury that we locked away for high days and holidays and was only consumed by the wealthy. Refined sugars simply didn't exist for our ancestors. Their diet consisted mainly of vegetables, fruit, cereals and some wild meat. It wasn't until this century that we developed an addiction to the sweet and sticky sugar family.

We clearly don't need refined sugar. What seems to have been overlooked is that our bodies can change complex carbohydrates and proteins into the sugar they require. Sugar contains no vitamins, no minerals, no protein, no fibre and no starches. It may contain tiny traces of calcium and magnesium if you're lucky, but primarily it provides us with loads of 'empty calories'.

It is actually a fair skill these days not to consume large amounts of sugar because it is added to so many foods. What do you think the following have in common? Cheese, biscuits, fruit yogurt, tomato sauce, baked beans, pickled cucumbers, muesli, beefburgers, Worcestershire sauce, pork sausages, peas, cornflakes and cola drinks – well, they can all contain sugar. Cola drinks contain some eight teaspoonfuls per can.

The nitty gritty about coffee

Over the last 10 years reports have begun to filter through about the health hazards attached to coffee, probably because increasing amounts of coffee are being consumed. Since 1950 the consumption of coffee in the UK has increased four-fold. Many people become quite addicted to it unknowingly, and can't give up the habit easily.

We now know that coffee aggravates nervous tension, anxiety and insomnia. So obviously, no matter how much we may enjoy it, drinking coffee to excess is not a healthy habit. In fact, coffee contains caffeine which is a mental and physical stimulant. This can be of benefit, of course, but even with two to four cups each day, adverse effects can be experienced. These include anxiety, restlessness, nervousness, insomnia, rapid pulse, palpitations, shakes and passing increased quantities of water. Regular coffee drinkers not only enjoy the flavour but in many cases come to rely on the stimulation to get them through the day. If you cannot get going without your first fix of the day, you will know what I mean!

Weaning yourself off coffee can sometimes be a fairly traumatic experience. It can sometimes produce symptoms not unlike a drug withdrawal, in particular a severe headache, which may take several days to disappear. However, rest assured, the headaches do eventually go completely, as long as you manage to abstain and use alternatives with which you are relatively happy.

How to kick the habit

- Cut down gradually over the space of a week or two.

- Use decaffeinated coffee instead, but limit yourself to two to three cups each day.

- Try alternative drinks like Barleycup, dandelion coffee or Bambu which you can obtain from health-food shops.

- If you like filter coffee, you can still use your filter, but with decaffeinated versions or with roasted dandelion root instead of coffee (get this from good health-food shops; it has a very pleasant malted flavour).

The truth about tea

The British are famous for their tea consumption. Tea, like coffee, contains caffeine, about 90 mg per mug, compared with coffee's 150 mg per mug. Tea also contains tannin, which inhibits the absorption of zinc and iron in particular. Excess tea produces the same effects as coffee and you can also experience withdrawal headaches. Tea can also cause constipation.

By drinking a cup of tea with a meal you can cut down the absorption of iron from vegetarian foods to one-third. Whereas a glass of fresh orange juice with the same meal would increase iron absorption by twice as much because of its high vitamin C content. Vegetarian and vegan women need their intake of iron to be readily absorbed, so drinking anything other than small amounts of weak tea may mean they risk becoming iron deficient.

'Herbal teas' don't count as tea as such. It's really a confusing name. Most herbal teas are free of caffeine and tannin and just consist of a collection of herbs. Unlike regular tea, they can be cleansing and relaxing. My favourite herbal tea 'look-alike' is Redbush herbal tea, which looks just like tea with milk but tastes even better. Many patients prefer it to ordinary tea, although it does take a week or two to get used to. It is available from most health-food shops.

More about alcohol

On average, women consume one unit of alcohol each day, and men three units (one unit = one glass of wine, one pub measure of spirits, one small sherry or vermouth, or half a pint of normal strength beer or lager). These average levels are now the maximum recommended daily intakes for women and men respectively. Although many of us may be teetotallers or drink substantially less than this, there will be those who regularly consume more. It is recognised that some women hit the bottle at the time of the menopause in an attempt to blot out reality.

Alcohol in excess destroys body tissue over the years and can cause or contribute to many diseases – for example, cardiovascular diseases, digestive disorders, inflammation and ulceration of the lining of the digestive tract, liver disease, brain degeneration, miscarriages, damage to unborn children and malnutrition. Last but not least, sustained heavy drinking can be a risk factor for osteoporosis.

As most of these conditions come on gradually, we often don't see the real dangers of alcohol. There is no impact like that of an accident or the drama of an ambulance arriving to carry you off. Instead, there is a slow process of destruction which conveniently escapes our awareness.

If you like your drink and notice that your consumption is becoming heavier because you feel low, you will be aware of the social problems that go with it, such as mood swings and personality changes. When this occurs, others around become affected and relationships may be strained at home and at work. It is a fact that one-third of the divorce petitions cite alcohol as a contributory factor. Local courtrooms are always having to deal with people who committed offences while under the influence of alcohol – so take stock.

Smoking

Smoking tobacco has become a widespread habit among Western societies. In 1922 in the UK, for example, 20- to 30-year-old women smoked an average of 50 cigarettes each year, but by 1975 this had risen to an average of just over 5,000 cigarettes per woman, per year. Although the more educated classes have reduced their cigarette consumption, smoking has become relatively common in those women who are less well educated.

It is generally acknowledged that women who regularly smoke in excess of 15 cigarettes each day are likely to have their menopause two years earlier than their non-smoking counterparts. Smoking also affects bone density; it should either be drastically cut down or, better still, stopped before the menopause.

Drugs

Western societies have become drug-oriented. In the USA in 1996 nearly $72 billion was spent on medicines by a population of 266 million, and in the UK it was £5.5 billion or around £100 per man, woman and child. Doctors issue some 15 per cent more prescriptions than they did a decade ago. In England alone, more than 473 million prescriptions were written in 1992, nearly 13.2 million for antidepressants, amounting to £147 million. None of this is surprising when you consider the power and influence that drug companies assume in the education of doctors.

In the last few years medical practitioners worldwide have been tremendously concerned about the excessive use of benzodiazepine tranquillisers and sleeping tablets. It is now recommended that these drugs, which include Valium, Mogadon and Ativan, are used as a temporary measure for only a few weeks. Those who have been taking them long-term should, if at all possible, have their dosage and frequency gradually reduced under medical supervision.

The quality of diet

Our diet this century has gone through, and continues to go through, several substantial changes. By the end of the 1970s there was evidence, from certain surveys, of a deterioration in the quality of the UK diet, particularly since the World War II. A high intake of sugar, refined foods, animal fats and alcohol had meant a relatively poor intake of essential vitamins and minerals.

Some 15 vitamins, 24 minerals and eight amino acids have been isolated as being essential for normal body function. They are synergistic, which means that they rely on each other in order to keep the body functioning at an optimum level. When one or more is in short supply, alterations in body metabolism occur. Minor deficiencies can often be tolerated, but major or multiple deficiencies result in the body becoming inefficient, with the development of symptoms and possibly disease.

There is, however, some heartening recent evidence. All the food advice from numerous individual experts and expert committees, government ones included, has finally got through to some of the British public. Many of us have increased our intake of fruit and vegetables and this greatly offsets the potential fall in intake from eating refined foods or eating smaller amounts of food in general. However, this has not happened with the unemployed or those who come from families where the main wage-earner is unskilled. From the recent dietary survey of British adults in the UK, the single biggest factor that determined nutrient intake was not age, sex, illness, or whether on a diet or not, but whether the person was unemployed. Like it or not, it seems that we already have a nutritional underclass who don't have the money and the knowledge to improve their diets. Fats and sugar are cheap calories and when you are hungry calories are more important than fibre, vitamins and minerals.

Water

Our most important nutrient is water, and sadly it is becoming one of our major sources of pollution. Not only is the water contaminated with lead, aluminium and copper, we now have nitrates to contend with as well. Nitrates are chemicals used in fertilisers to promote crop growth. These are harmful because they go through a chemical change and at the end of the day turn into nitrosamines which are believed to be strong cancer-producing chemicals.

Lead and other toxic minerals

Toxic minerals in the form of lead and mercury are in the soil, the air and the water, as well as being present in our food. During this century their levels have been rising rapidly, at times to a point where our bodies have not been able to cope.

Lead pollution has been much discussed in the media over the past few years. High lead levels are acknowledged to be linked to low birth weight and low intelligence in children. As a result of extensive research on lead, many countries have removed lead from petrol and are trying to keep lead levels down in cities. However, it is far more difficult to remove it from the water supply as the filtering systems at water-purification plants can't always cope with the load.

How to avoid toxins

- Concentrate on eating a nutritious diet, particularly high in zinc, magnesium, calcium and vitamins C, B and E (see also page 112).
- Take a well-balanced multivitamin supplement and some extra vitamin C if you are at particular risk.

107

- Scrub all fruit and vegetables with a brush to clean off as many toxins as possible, and remove the outer layers of lettuce and cabbage, etc. But don't *peel* fruit and vegetables unless you don't like the peel – very often the bulk of the nutrients is just under the skin. Buy organic vegetables and salad stuff or grow your own where possible, without using chemicals.
- Water filters tend to filter out many of the toxic metals. Every so often the filter needs replacing and it's amazing what collects in it. Rather the toxic deposits collect in the filter than in your body! Water purifiers can be bought in healthfood shops but they aren't so efficient.
- Do not spend too much time near busy roads if the local exhaust fumes contain lead (which may be easier said than done).
- Avoid copper and aluminium cookware unless it has a non-stick lining.
- Cut down on alcohol, as it increases lead absorption.
- Do not eat refined foods: these give the body little protection against toxins.
- Avoid antacids which contain aluminium salts.

Food additives

While some perfectly harmless substances are added to food, the number of potentially harmful additives is significant. Many additives have been shown to cause hyperactivity in children, as well as asthma, eczema, skin rashes and swelling. It's obviously important to be able to differentiate between the safe and the not-so-safe additives.

After being bombarded by warnings about additives, is it any wonder that some of us have at one time or another avoided all foods containing them? Understandably, 'additive' has become a dirty word in some circles. But it's important to understand that some additives are, in fact, beneficial! For example, beneficial additives include riboflavin – vitamin B2 – and calcium L-ascorbate, which is vitamin C, and the many preservatives which help to keep our food from spoiling. Look in Appendix 3 on page 319 for details of booklets and books on additives which will help you to distinguish the dangerous additives from the safe ones.

TAKE ONE POSITIVE STEP AT A TIME

I am sorry to bombard you with so many depressing facts all at once. We, the consumers, definitely need more information about the food we eat and the environmental factors to which we are subjected.

Probably the first step towards reversing the effects of the 21st century on your body is for you to acknowledge the value of that body if you haven't already done so. After all, you only have one body to last you the rest of your life, so it's important to treat it with respect.

It's up to you how often you expose your body to alcohol, cigarettes, drugs and harmful additives, and how physically fit you keep through exercise. Making one change at a time is better than not changing at all.

If you have been neglecting your body to some extent, now may be the time to make some changes. Don't expect your doctor to piece you back together again when you have fallen apart through 'environmental wear and nutritional tear'! It's up to each one of us to look after our bodies to the best of our abilities and to treat them as well as any other of our treasured possessions.

As for environmental pollution, there are now many worthwhile national and local groups running campaigns to help to overcome these problems. You will find a list of these in Appendix 4 on page 324. If you are concerned about your local situation, you can always contact your area government representative for help and advice.

7

NUTRITION AND HORMONE FUNCTION

There is now no doubt that our diet influences our hormone function. Medical researchers are beginning to work it out for women and eventually they will also work it out for men. So far it would seem that our hormonal balance is determined by diet and nutritional state in three ways:

- The balance of fat and fibre in the diet
- The effects of individual essential nutrients
- The presence of natural oestrogen and progesterone compounds in foodstuffs (see Chapter 8).

Before we launch into these three areas, we must first acknowledge that we do not actually know how important these components are. It is safe to say that they have been overlooked and their importance will rise perhaps to a point where dietary change will be acknowledged for some women, by Uncle Tom Cobley and all, as a real alternative to HRT for the control of oestrogen-withdrawal symptoms. That is our impression from many of the women we have seen and advised in a clinic setting.

We are not talking about diet and osteoporosis. That is a quite different topic and it is covered in Chapter 9.

FAT AND FIBRE

This duo, who took leading roles in the story of heart disease, have also been busy at work on the rise and fall of oestrogen. Scientific interest primarily came about because of the strong relationship between dietary intake of fat, and heart disease and breast cancer. Those countries with a high intake of fat, especially saturated fat found predominantly in animal products, have a high rate of breast cancer. As yet we do not know whether reducing our intake of fat will reduce the rate of breast cancer. Such studies would be costly and complicated and have not yet been undertaken. What has been studied is the influence of our diet and its fat and fibre content on hormone function and the possible attendant risks of breast disease. Some of this information is of relevance when trying to understand the relationship between diet and hormone changes at the menopause.

In brief, the majority of studies have shown that:

- A high-fat, low-fibre diet is associated with relatively high levels of circulating oestrogen
- Dietary fibre enhances the rate of clearance of oestrogen from the body
- In premenopausal women, changing to a low-fat, high-fibre diet can, but does not always, lower the circulating oestrogen levels
- Vegetarians and those who are not overweight tend to have higher levels of a hormone-modifying protein: sex hormone binding globulin (SHBG), in their blood. This helps to smooth out the highs and lows of hormone function
- Severe constipation is associated with a high level of oestrogen and menstrual irregularities
- By killing off friendly bacteria in the intestine, antibiotics may reduce the natural recycling of oestrogen by the body.

What this jumble of information indicates is not fully clear. In essence, the extremes of diet and bowel function are associated with the more extreme levels of hormones, especially oestrogen. A lifelong high-fat, low-fibre diet is more likely to be associated with menopausal symptoms of oestrogen withdrawal. This may be because these women's systems are used to a relatively high level of circulating hormones so they tolerate the drop less well. In theory, making a dramatic change to a low-fat, high-fibre diet might aggravate the symptoms of oestrogen withdrawal in women in the perimenopause or early postmenopause. This effect is likely to be offset by the impact of improved nutrition on hormone function.

In summary, there seems to be an excessive hormonal vulnerability in those consuming a Western diet. Make the change but do not be too drastic about it at the time of the menopause: for example, don't suddenly go from being a meat-eater to following a weight-loss vegan diet! Changing your diet may help not only to reduce the risks of heart disease, but also the risks of the hormonally related cancers in the breast and womb.

INDIVIDUAL ESSENTIAL NUTRIENTS

It appears that many nutrients are essential either for the production of hormones or to help the way in which the hormones do their job in the body. Nutritional deficiencies have to be severe before they have a profound influence, but several combined nutritional inadequacies will probably have a subtle adverse effect on hormone function. You may think that nutritional deficiencies are rare in the UK. True, if we confine ourselves to severe deficiencies. But from authoritative government surveys, poor intake of a number of nutrients are acknowledged in some 20 per cent of women of child-bearing age. So there is absolutely no room for nutritional complacency.

Let's take an individual look at some of the important nutrients.

Iron

The main function of iron is the production of the oxygen-carrying blood pigment haemoglobin. Iron is also needed by muscles and the brain, and a lack causes not only anaemia but also fatigue, loss of hair and brittle, split nails. Anaemia occurs in 4 per cent of women of child-bearing age but has to be severe to result in cessation of periods. Mild lack of iron is more likely and can be present in a further 10 per cent of the menstruating population. It can cause fatigue and should be considered in any perimenopausal woman in whom this is a problem.

Vitamin B

There are several members of the vitamin B family. Broadly speaking, they are involved in energy release from food and the health of the nervous system. Severe deficiency of two of these vitamins is on record as causing cessation of menstruation or menstrual irregularities. These are vitamin B12 and vitamin B3. Deficiencies of either of these is rare.

Lack of vitamin B12 can occur in long-standing strict vegans and in older people who lose the ability to absorb this vitamin. Weight loss, fatigue, tingling in the feet and loss of balance are other features of this deficiency.

Lack of vitamin B3 – nicotinic acid or niacinamide – should only develop in the heavy alcohol consumer, those on very poor low-protein diets and those with serious digestive problems. Depression, a red, scaly rash on the face, backs of the hands or other light-exposed areas and diarrhoea are other features. In malnourished women deficient in this vitamin, menstrual irregularities were apparently common. It might occasionally be a problem in the perimenopausal woman if she is drinking rather heavily.

Vitamin B6 is often linked with premenstrual syndrome. Mild deficiency diagnosed by a low blood level is surprisingly common and together with lack of vitamin B1, thiamin, is known to be a common finding in both men and women with anxiety and depression. Deficiency of this, however, is not known to be associated with any menstrual disturbance. Vitamin B6, however, is involved in the way in which tissues respond to oestrogen and is apparently needed for that part on the surface of the cell that interacts with oestrogen to refresh itself. Hence increased amounts of vitamin B6 may be needed by some women who are taking relatively large amounts of oestrogen, as in the oral contraceptive pill. HRT seems to have a much less disturbing effect in this respect. It is theoretically possible that the response of tissues to oestrogen would be improved by correction of a vitamin B6 deficiency or by taking an extra amount of it.

Though severe lack of these and the other B vitamins are fairly infrequent, mild deficiency is not that uncommon even in relatively well-fed populations. Such has been the concern about the poor intake of folic acid in women of child-bearing age that, since December 1992, all women in the UK who wish to become pregnant are now advised to take a daily supplement of 400 micrograms, nearly twice the average dietary intake, before conceiving. Doing so greatly reduces the chance of the mother giving birth to an infant with spina bifida. There may well be other adverse effects of mild vitamin B deficiency in women of child-bearing age that are not yet documented. Menstrual disturbance is one possibility.

Vitamin E

The use of Vitamin E in women of reproductive age was stimulated by the early discovery that in rats, deficiency caused pregnant females to abort and lose their offspring. Indeed, the proper chemical name for vitamin E is tocopherol, which in Greek means child-bearing. In premenstrual women, in fact women with premenstrual syndrome, supplements of vitamin E have been found to raise oestrogen levels but the response varied considerably with the dose. Its effect on hormone chemistry in perimenopausal and postmenopausal women has unfortunately not been studied. However, its effect on hot flushes has been recorded since 1949. In the earliest study a response rate of over 50 per cent was recorded when high doses, in the region of 1,000 IUs per day were given. Although the trial was not scientific enough to convince today's doctors, this early report included the case of one woman who resumed menstruation ten months after she had received radiation treatment to destroy her ovaries. So we cannot rule it out completely. Again, we would like to know if some menopausal women have a relative lack of this vitamin. Lower-than-average levels have been associated with a higher-than-average risk of breast cancer. So it might help some women: perhaps those in the perimenopause rather than those who are truly postmenstrual.

We often use vitamin E as part of our programme for menopausal women: try 200 IUs initially each day.

Magnesium

This mineral has come from obscurity to the verge of fame in the last ten years. The cousin of calcium, it is necessary for normal bone, muscle and nerve function. It is also the sister of potassium and like her is found mainly inside cells controlling energy functions. Good sources of potassium are fresh fruit and vegetables, especially green ones. From dietary assessments it appears that between 10 and 20 per cent of women of child-bearing age consume less than the minimum recommended amounts of these nutrients.

Magnesium and some other minerals are also involved in hormone function. Experiments have shown that this mineral is needed by the ovaries in order for them to respond satisfactorily to the stimulatory effect of the pituitary hormones, LH and FSH. The failure to respond to them on the part of the ovaries is exactly what happens at the menopause. We don't think that lack of magnesium is the cause of the menopause! However, it does often seem to be moderately lacking in women of all ages with premenstrual syndrome; and we know that supplements of it can help PMS. So it wouldn't be too surprising if it was having some influence over some menopausal problems. Good candidates would include an early menopause, erratic cycles, fatigue, depression and aches and pains.

A high-magnesium diet is very nutritious and supplements are harmless enough; the only likely side-effect is diarrhoea which, for those who are constipated, might be a help. No studies, as yet, have looked at the relationship between magnesium and either the timing or the symptoms of the menopause. From our own experience we have seen a rather variable picture when we have looked at the results of red-cell magnesium levels, which are known to be low in 50 per cent of women with PMS and do seem to be low in some women with menopausal difficulties. Again, it is asking too much to blame everything on to one nutrient; what is needed are large studies that look at nutritional factors in detail. We have found a magnesium and calcium supplement called Gynovite useful in treating hot flushes, and it may also encourage bone regeneration.

« Madelaine's Story *»*

Madelaine was thirty-five when she had one of her ovaries removed because of a large cyst. Eleven years later, her periods were becoming irregular and even though she was not experiencing hot flushes she wondered if she might be approaching the menopause. Along with her periods, of which she had had six in the preceding twelve months, she was experiencing migraine headaches, breast tenderness and lumps, and fluid retention. The breast tenderness had been partly helped by Efamol Evening Primrose Oil.

Investigations showed significantly increased levels of the hormones FSH and LH into the 'menopausal range'. Nutritional tests showed low levels of vitamin B, magnesium and essential fatty acids of both the vegetable and fish-oil types, so it was therefore possible that Madelaine's hormone function was being compromised by her nutritional state.

A change in her diet was suggested to reduce the intake of saturated animal fats and to increase her intake of the polyunsaturated essential fats. Foods known to be common triggers of migraine were also to be avoided, as were salt and salty foods. Supplements of multivitamins, magnesium and evening primrose oil with fish oils were recommended to be taken for several months. These measures resulted in a reduction of her migraine headaches and a substantial lessening of her breast problems.

Initially there was no influence on her periods and it seemed likely that HRT might well be necessary. After four months she had three periods at three- to four-week intervals and after a further eight-week gap there then followed a further four periods, all at regular intervals. The period-associated symptoms had all diminished greatly and the need for HRT had seemed to fade. In fact, a repeat of the hormone tests showed a substantial fall in the levels of FSH and LH to premenopausal levels, supporting the notion that Madelaine's ovaries were responding more easily to the cyclical stimulation from the pituitary. The previously deficient nutrients had also improved.

This is an example of how attention to nutritional problems in the perimenopause might influence the regularity of the menstrual cycle and the symptoms associated with it.

Zinc

This mineral is certainly important for men, as even a mild lack of it, if prolonged, can have a profound effect on sperm and testosterone production. By rights it should be important to women but we do not know of any evidence to this effect. Intakes in the UK are pretty close to the minimum recommended amounts and absorption is easily reduced by alcohol, bran and many other foods. The best dietary source is Atlantic oysters followed by beef and most other meats (so you know what to give him for dinner tonight). It would probably take a severe lack to upset hormone function and this is only likely in the heavy alcohol consumer and those eating a low-protein diet.

Essential fatty acids

Some fats, like vitamins and minerals, are essential. These essential fats are the polyunsaturates found in most vegetable oils and oily fish. We've heard a lot about them in heart disease and the story doesn't end there. They are not easy things to study. First, your body only needs a tiny amount of them, which is just as well as that's all it usually gets with our modern-day diet. A deficiency builds up over years, possibly decades, before it takes its toll. We know so far that severe deficiency is rare and is confined to premature infants, alcoholics (again) and the malnourished. A mild or relative deficiency can develop in the 'normal' population and this could be a factor in heart disease. Intakes and blood levels generally fall with increasing age.

On the hormone front, essential fatty acids are doing something very interesting. These fats are used in the building of cell walls and in particular seem to influence the function of those pieces of cell machinery that are actually embedded in the cell wall, such as the receptors for hormones. Complicated but interesting. So it is possible that a relative lack of these essential fatty acids over many years might modify the way in which our bodies respond to certain hormones. So what's the evidence? Well, in the cheetah a lack of the essential fishy fatty acids, particularly of the omega-3 series, results in infertility because of an inability of the female to ovulate. Sounds familiar? And in the human? Sorry, right now we don't know but again it's a possible factor. Certain specialized preparations of these essential fatty acids have already been of demonstrable benefit in a variety of diverse areas. So far we have seen Efamol evening primrose oil (the omega-6 series) benefit women with premenstrual breast tenderness and also help some adults and children with dry eczema.

The fish oils have also made their mark in reducing the pain and inflammation of rheumatoid arthritis and they help to lower elevated levels of some blood fats – not cholesterol. A number of studies suggest that combining calcium with essential fatty acids from evening primrose oil and marine fish oil, may be an effective way of preventing osteoporosis. A recently published study, conducted by Dr Kruger and her colleagues from the University of Pretoria, South Africa, tested the effect of these oils on calcium balance in a group of women with osteoporosis. After a four-month trial period, there were a number of changes which suggested increased absorption of calcium from the diet and increased uptake of calcium by the bone.

The efficacy of this combination was discovered through a number of known factors:

- The Inuits (formerly known as Eskimos) rarely develop renal stones. This is thought to be due to the high dietary content of marine oils reducing the spillage of calcium into the urine. Recently Mr Colin Buck and colleagues from Glasgow Royal Infirmary used essential fatty acid supplements to treat patients who developed kidney stones due to the excessive loss of calcium in the urine. The combination of Efamol evening primrose oil and marine fish oil was particularly effective in reducing urinal loss of calcium and, interestingly, increased the absorption of calcium from the diet.
- Drugs given to babies with heart disease that alter chemical processes related to essential fatty acids also cause rapid bone development.
- Lack of essential fatty acids reduces the effectiveness of vitamin D in animals, resulting in weaker bones.
- Subsequent careful studies have established the best combination of evening primrose oil and marine oil, which encourages calcium absorption and reduces calcium loss in the urine. This combination is known as Efacal (from Efamol), and each capsule of Efacal contains 400 mg of Efamol pure evening primrose oil, 44 mg of marine fish oil and 100 mg of calcium.

Efacal has been shown to:

- Improve the uptake of calcium from the diet through the gut wall;
- Decrease the amount of calcium lost through the urine;
- Help direct calcium to sites of deposition in the bone and may thus help prevent the bone-thinning process. It is effectively the stamp on the envelope that makes delivery far more likely.

The essential fatty acids are all going to have other uses too but it would seem that their full benefit will only be realized if they are taken long-term for months, possibly years, and are accompanied by a very healthy diet rich in these same oils. And any associated deficiencies of vitamins and minerals need to be corrected, as they too influence the chemistry of these fats; and any underlying disease, like diabetes, for example, also needs to be treated. So it is not a quick fix.

Choosing your nutritional supplements

If you plan to take nutritional supplements you will need to choose them with care. We don't advise women to take random supplements without first seeking proper advice. Our bodies are fairly sensitive mechanisms with specific needs and too much of any one particular nutrient can cause imbalances which may lead to other problems in the long-term.

Before choosing your supplements, take a look at the chart below on the physical signs of nutritional deficiency. You may recognize some deficiency which you have had for years, but have accepted as being 'normal'.

Physical signs of vitamin and mineral deficiency

Sign or symptom	Can be caused by deficiencies of
Cracking at the corners of the mouth	Iron, vitamins B12, B6, Folic acid
Recurrent mouth ulcers	Iron, vitamins B12, B6, Folic acid
Dry, cracked lips	Vitamin B2
Smooth (sore) tongue	Iron, vitamins B2, B12, Folic acid
Enlargement/prominence of taste buds at tip of tongue (red, sore)	Vitamins B2, or B6
Red, greasy skin on face, especially sides of nose	Vitamins B2, B6, zinc or essential fatty acids
Rough, sometimes red, pimply skin on upper arms and thighs	Vitamin B complex, vitamin E or essential fatty acids
Skin conditions such as eczema, dry, rough, cracked, peeling skin	Zinc, essential fatty acids
Poor hair growth	Iron or zinc
Dandruff	Vitamin C, vitamin B6, zinc, essential fatty acids
Acne	Zinc
Bloodshot, gritty, sensitive eyes	Vitamins A or B2
Night blindness	Vitamin A or zinc

Sign or symptom	Can be caused by deficiencies of
Dry eyes	Vitamin A, essential fatty acids
Brittle or split nails	Iron, zinc or essential fatty acids
Pale appearance due to anaemia	Iron, vitamin B12, Folic acid, essential to consult your doctor

Depending on the symptoms you are currently suffering, there are several useful supplements that can be tried in conjunction with each other. Assuming your symptoms are severe and that you are looking for the most effective treatment, I shall first suggest the optimum regime to begin with, regardless of cost. I shall then go on to discuss cheaper alternatives.

Vitamin and mineral supplements

The best all-round option is to take a multivitamin and mineral supplement which contains good amounts of the essential nutrients mentioned. The supplement we favour, which has been through a clinical trial, is called Gynovite. It was formulated by Dr Guy Abraham in the USA and is the sister preparation to Optivite, the clinically tried and tested supplement for PMS. In the UK it is available from health-food shops and by mail order from Nutritional Health (address on page 120). For severe symptoms you will need to take between four and six tablets each day, ideally splitting the dose between breakfast and lunch. Work up to the full dose gradually over a week or two. If your symptoms are moderate, you could probably manage with between two and three tablets each day.

Efacal is a specially formulated new product, produced by Efamol, which contains evening primrose oil, marine fish oil and calcium. It has been designed as a daily supplement and comes in capsule form. There is some medical evidence to show that supplements containing calcium are more likely to be effectively absorbed when taken in the evening.

Those at risk of osteoporosis should take four capsules every day with the evening meal. *For preventative purposes,* four capsules should be taken every day for an initial twelve-week period, followed by a daily dose of two capsules.

Once you have selected your basic supplement, you will need to add other appropriate products. Read through the chart below and decide which extra supplements you need. Where two or more options are listed for one set of symptoms, try one of the supplements under that heading first. If after a few months you are not convinced that it is helping, switch to the alternative. As we are all so individual, we may respond to different supplements, so it is sometimes a matter of trial and error. Keep a note of what you try on your personal programme chart on page 215.

Matching supplement to symptom

Problem	Type of supplement	Daily dosage	Available from
Hot flushes and	*Novogen Red Clover	1 40 mg tablet	Health food shops and WNAS
nightsweats	*Natural vitamin E	200–400 IUs	Boots, chemist, Health food shops and Nutritional Health
	Panax ginseng	1–2 600 mg capsules	Health food shops
	4:40 Plus (vitamin E + ginseng)	1–2 600 mg capsules	Chemist, health food shops
Anxiety, irritability, or mood swings, depression	*Gynovite	2–4 tablets	Health food shops or WNAS
Libido	*Hypericum (St John's wort)	300 mg with each meal	Chemists, health food shops or WNAS
Eczema, dry skin	*Efamol/Epogam	2–8 500 IU capsules	Boots, chemists or WNAS
Heavy periods	*Gynovite	Dose as above	As above
	Iron-ferrous sulphate	1 200 mg tablet with fruit juice	Chemists
Painful periods	*Magnesium amino acid chelate	2–4 150 mg tablets at night	Health food shops or WNAS
Breast tenderness	*Efamol/Efamast	As above	Boots, chemists, health food shops or WNAS
Constipation	*Magnesium amino acid chelate	2–5 150 mg tablets at night	Health food shops or WNAS
	Linusit Gold	2 tablespoons	Health food shops
Osteoporosis	Calcium carbonate, gluconate or citrate	1000 mg of elemental calcium	Chemists and health food shops
	*Magnesium amino acid chelate	150–600 mg elemental magnesium	Health food shops and WNAS
	*Efacal (Ostical NZ)	4 capsules daily (preferably taken at night)	Boots, chemists, and health food shops

* Available by mail order through Women's Nutritional Advisory Service, PO Box 268, Lewes, East Sussex BN7 1QN

Important points

- Never take supplements without the consent of your GP if you have a current medical problem.
- Always begin taking your supplements gradually. For example, if you are due to take two or four of a particular supplement each day, begin taking one tablet each day and gradually build up to the optimum dosage over a week or two. Take them after meals unless otherwise specified.

Should you keep taking the supplements for ever?
If you have decided not to take HRT, or can't take it for any reason, apart from wanting to control your symptoms associated with the menopause, you will need to prevent osteoporosis in the long-term. For this reason, more than any other, continue to take supplements that include evening primrose oil, marine fish oil and calcium for as long as you can. You are most at risk of bone-loss for the five years following the menopause, and although the loss slows down in the following ten years, it is still pretty significant. We recommend eating well, doing weight-bearing exercise and taking a moderate dose of supplements in the long term.

What about drugs?
If you are taking prescribed drugs from your doctor, you are not advised to stop taking them or to reduce them without his or her consent. However, we do find that, once established on their holistic programme, many women no longer feel the need for their tranquillizers, antidepressants or sleeping pills. Nutritional supplements can be taken quite happily alongside most drugs, as can HRT. There are a few exceptions, however. Any antibiotic in the tetracycline family should not be taken with a supplement of minerals. Evening primrose oil should not be taken by anyone with epilepsy. When you feel the time has come to reduce your drugs, do go to see your doctor for a discussion before taking any action, especially if you have been taking them for a long time. Coming off drugs suddenly may bring on nasty withdrawal symptoms so make it a gradual process.

8

THE PHYTOESTROGEN FACTOR

It is not widely appreciated that Mother Nature, in her wisdom, has given us a number of plant foods which are rich in naturally occurring oestrogens. These phytoestrogens, as they are known, can provide us with a constant source of oestrogen, if we know where to look for them. Found in small quantities in plants ('phyto' means 'plant' in Greek), they help to maintain falling oestrogen levels at the time of the menopause and, as a bonus, protect us against heart disease and the bone-thinning disease, osteoporosis.

Phytoestrogens are good news for us all, but particularly for women from mid-life onwards. They are a family of naturally occurring substances with a chemical structure very similar to our own female hormone, oestrogen. Although similar in structure to oestrogen, they are much less potent. Despite this, research shows that they protect us against hormonally related cancers and have the ability to block the uptake of excess oestrogen by the body, and even raise low levels when necessary.

The Japanese language, until recently, did not include the term 'hot flush', largely because Japanese women, who consume a diet rich in phytoestrogens, hardly experience any adverse symptoms at the time of the menopause, that is until they deviate from their traditional diet.

THE IMPORTANCE OF OESTROGEN

Although the hormone oestrogen was first identified in the late 1920s, it is only in recent years that many of its important functions have come to be appreciated amongst medical communities. These include:

- Playing an important role in the formation of the reproductive organs of males and females
- Regulating menstrual cycles and pregnancies

- Reducing the risk of heart disease and the bone-thinning disease osteoporosis
- Keeping skin, hair and nails in good shape.

THE POWER OF PHYTOESTROGENS

A wealth of research in recent years has demonstrated that a phyto-estrogen-rich diet can perform 'medical miracles'. Apart from being able dramatically to reduce hot flushes and other oestrogen withdrawal symptoms at the time of the menopause, phytoestrogens have been shown to have many other abilities, including:

- Turning cancer cells back into normal healthy cells
- Unblocking clogged arteries
- Significantly reducing LDL, the bad cholesterol and raising HDL, the good cholesterol
- Helping to generate new bone, thus protecting our bones against osteoporosis
- Normalising blood sugar, thus helping to control diabetes
- Helping to regulate the menstrual cycle.

Despite all this, and the fact that there are thousands of medical studies published on this subject, carried out by conventional researchers around the world, phytoestrogens are little known outside medical and nutritional research circles. The vast majority of doctors completely underestimate the impact dietary factors can have on our health.

THE FOUR MAIN TYPES OF PHYTOESTROGENS

New research is clearly beginning to demonstrate the individual strengths of the most common phytoestrogens, and it is becoming apparent which cells in the body have affinity for the different forms. As time goes by, the names of the most recognised phytoestrogens will become part of our everyday language, so let us examine them.

Genistein is the most extensively studied isoflavone to date and, although it was identified as a plant oestrogen in 1966, its anti-cancer properties were not recognised by medical researchers for another 20 years. Japanese researchers first discovered that genistein, found in soy products, was capable of blocking the signal that triggers the growth of a cancer cell, and that it was also able to inhibit the growth of a cancerous tumour.

Daidzein, the second major phytoestrogen to be discovered, like genistein acts as both an anti-cancer agent and an antioxidant. It also has a role to play in the prevention of bone mass depletion and is able to cause cancer cells to revert to normal.

Formononetin and Biochanin A are two more recently discovered oestrogenic isoflavones which are chiefly derived from Red Clover, chickpeas, lentils and mung beans. Formononetin is a methylated daidzein, and boichanin a methylated genistein. They have unique effects on human physiology that are not possessed by the non-methylated isoflavones genistein and daidzein found in soya. As well as being cancer-protective compounds, they are also responsible for the positive lipid (blood fat) lowering properties associated with traditional diets.

Lignans like soy products, possess both weak oestrogenic and anti-oestrogenic qualities, and are structurally similar to oestradiol, a form of oestrogen. In humans, lignans are derived mainly from linseeds, converted by intestinal bacteria to hormone-like compounds. When organic linseeds are consumed, Linusit Gold, intestinal bacterial action results in the production of up to eight hundred times more of these lignans from any other food. They have a positive effect on sex hormone production, metabolism, growth, biological and enzyme function, and to some degree, have a protective effect against some forms of cancer, particularly breast cancer. They also have antifungal, antibacterial and antiviral properties.

HOW DO PHYTOESTROGENS WORK?

It seems that they are able to compete with oestrogens within the body and the harmful environmental oestrogens (xenoestrogens) for the receptor sites at the entrance to the cells. So, for example, genistein, the look-alike oestrogen, is successfully able to take up occupation in breast tissue, thus preventing the more potent oestrogen from converting normal cells into cancer cells. Because genistein is able to block the uptake of oestrogen, it acts as an 'anti-oestrogen', in a similar way to the drug tamoxifen administered to breast cancer victims, but without the side-effects.

Phytoestrogens are fast becoming known as great hormone regulators, in that they can both increase and decrease the levels of oestrogen in the body, depending upon the circumstances. When oestrogen is in oversupply in the body, as can occur prior to the menopause, phyto-estrogens play 'musical chairs' with oestrogen in competition for the receptor sites within the cells. Some of the phytoestrogens will inevitably displace oestrogen, and because they are many times weaker in their effect, they reduce the cancer-promoting effects of the hormone proper. Phytoestrogens also dilute the effects of environmental oestrogen (xenoestrogens) which can be even more harmful to the body than normal oestrogens. On the other hand, if you are producing too little oestrogen, for example at the time of the menopause and beyond, phytoestrogens can give levels a natural boost, thus helping to combat symptoms such as hot flushes and osteoporosis.

Much more exciting research has since been conducted on the effects of phytoestrogens to the point where it has been discovered that they have certain similarities to the 'designer hormones', the Selective Oestrogen Receptor Modulators (SERMS) whereby they are able to bind to cells in certain parts of the body, without having a dramatic effect on others. This group of hormones is being developed to retain their beneficial effects on the cardiovascular system and the skeleton, without having cancer-promoting effects on the breasts or the lining of the womb. However, unlike phytoestrogens which help to relieve hot flushes, the down side with the SERMS is that they seem to cause hot flushes!

WHAT THE RESEARCH SHOWS

I first encountered phytoestrogens in 1990, when I read, in the *British Medical Journal*, about some research that had been conducted by Australian doctors. They had put a group of menopausal women who were not undergoing HRT on a diet rich in soy products, organic lin-seeds and a herb called Red Clover, all of which are rich in naturally occurring oestrogens. They demonstrated that it was possible to bring about the same changes in the lining of the vagina in these women as experienced by women undergoing HRT. This was great news for the 'alternative' camp, proving that naturally occurring oestrogens can be as effective as HRT.

A validation of how effective phytoestrogens may be was subsequently published in *The Lancet* in 1992. The study concluded that Japanese women do not seem to experience hot flushes and other menopausal symptoms because the Japanese diet contains foods rich in plant oestrogens, such as soy products and ginseng.

Since that time, there have been many positive studies published on phytoestrogens and their role in controlling the oestrogen-with-drawal symptoms of menopause. I have selected a few key studies that will be of great interest. In 1996, for example, researchers at the Royal Hospital for Women in New South Wales published a review on the clinical effects of phytoestrogens. They identified 861 relevant articles that reached positive conclusions about the associated health benefits.

Another study on phytoestrogens and the menopause, conducted by researchers at the University of South Manchester in England, also found positive results. They fed menopausal women a 60-gram soy protein drink daily for two months, and were able to reduce hot flushes by half, and the remaining flushes were 30 per cent less severe. Another soy protein experiment was set up by Professor Burke, of the department of public health science at the Bowman Gray School of Medicine, Winston-Salem, North Carolina. He fed 43 American women, aged between 45 and 55, 20 grams of soy protein, sprinkled over their morning cereal, for six weeks. They found that symptoms significantly reduced, although they did not entirely disappear. So they now have a larger ongoing study, with much higher doses of soy.

In 1998 Dr Albertuzzi confirmed the value of soy protein in helping to control hot flushes. In his study, 104 post-menopausal women took either 72 mg of isoflavones or a placebo each day for 12 weeks. Results showed that soy was significantly superior in reducing the number of hot flushes experienced. Women taking soy decreased their hot flushes by 26 per cent after three weeks, 33 per cent by week four, and 45 per cent by week 12, compared with a 30 per cent reduction in the hot flushes of women in the placebo group. Amazingly, some of the tested foods contained hardly any phytoestrogens. The phytoestrogen content of food may vary considerably depending on the crop, the time of year it was grown, the climate, and a number of environmental factors. Foods that have been put through scientific analysis will state the phytoestrogen content on the label, so once again it is down to label reading, or alternatively you could bake some of the bread, fruit loaves, cakes or biscuits that are detailed in the recipe section, beginning on page 300, and additionally in my book *The Phyto Factor* (see page 321).

A few years ago, an Australian study of menopausal women consuming bread rich in both soy and linseeds, showed a 40 per cent reduction in hot flushes and a small increase in bone mass. This preliminary research indicates that these phytoestrogens may well be as powerful as HRT, not just in their effect on vaginal tissue, but also in protecting us against both osteoporosis and heart disease. The soy and linseed loaf is now available in the UK in the form of the Burgen Loaf and Vogel Soy & Linseed loaf, available in supermarkets, in Australia as the Burgen Soy-Lin Loaf and in New Zealand as Country Fare Soya and Linseed Bread. The availability of this new bread, like the Burgen Loaf, makes it easier for many women in the Western world to include phytoestrogens in their diet on a regular basis, without having to change their eating habits. Four slices per day of these loaves are equivalent to a typical Oriental or Asian daily serving of phytoestrogens. Other foods rich in plant oestrogens are now finding their way onto the market, including snack bars, drinks and desserts. At the WNAS we have just had our Phyto Muesli made up into retail packs as it has proved such a popular 'phyto fix' with our patients. Naturally, as the research in this area is so positive, we will find many other products on our shelves in the very near future. We need to be discerning, however, as many foods may well contain phytoestrogen-rich ingredients in principle, but it is very difficult to standardise food as evidenced by the results of a survey conducted by Novogen in Australia. They analysed a long list of common phytoestrogen-rich foods, including soy products, chickpeas and lentils, and found a terrific variation of phytoestrogen content.

So, Mother Nature has provided us with foods that allow us to top up quite naturally on our oestrogen levels at the time of the menopause and beyond, without having to resort to Hormone Replacement Therapy. The only problem seems to be that women are generally unaware of which foods contain phytoestrogens. For details about how to incorporate these plant foods into your diet, follow the instructions in Parts Three and Four, beginning on pages 144 and 207 respectively.

CAN WE OVERDOSE ON PHYTOESTROGENS?

Although studies have used up to 160 mg of isoflavones daily for three months and recorded positive effects, the long-term effect of high doses has not been studied. As the average Asian diet delivers between 50 and 100 mg of isoflavones per day, it would seem reasonable not to exceed this dose. This matches the level that has been found to have a therapeutic effect in several clinical trials, and therefore seems a good compromise. The suggested menus in both this book and The Phyto Factor, have been designed to deliver up to 100 mg of isoflavones per day.

WHAT ABOUT MEN AND CHILDREN?

Asian men consume between 40 and 70 mg of isoflavones daily and have done so for centuries, without, it seems, any adverse health effects. In fact, scientists believe that men have a reduced death rate from both prostate cancer and heart disease as a result of their phytoestrogen consumption. Asian children also consume phytoestrogens daily, once again without any adverse health report. Professor Kenneth Setchell, who has probably conducted more research on phytoestrogens than any other researcher in the world, believes that the earlier the exposure to phytoestrogens the better.

WHAT ABOUT NATURAL PROGESTERONE?

There is some theoretic evidence to support the concept that progesterone is important in bone health, and this may apply to natural progesterone and some other synthetic preparations. Large doses of synthetic progesterone, together with calcium, have been reported to reduce the rate of bone loss in elderly men receiving steroids. Markers of progesterone adequacy in women, such as length of menstrual cycle, do seem to correlate with the rate of bone loss in premenopausal women. The rate of bone loss in premenopausal women also appeared to be related to the level of progesterone in the body.

Dr John Lee has reported that the use of natural progesterone, in the form of a cream applied to the skin which is derived from wild yam and marketed as Progest, can produce improvements in bone mineral density. The women he has studied were also advised to take supplements of calcium and magnesium and make changes to their diet. It is impossible to know at this stage from research published so far, until a trial on progesterone alone has been undertaken, which was the most effective or most important element of his studies. Progesterone could have a modifying influence on the rate of bone loss and the symptoms of oestrogen withdrawal – hot flushes and nightsweats – at the time of the menopause. Before using progesterone it is advisable to be tested to see whether a progesterone deficiency is actually present. Progest is only available on prescription.

It has been shown that women suffering from premenstrual syndrome, and with a slightly reduced progesterone level, can raise these levels by improving their diet and by taking a magnesium-rich multivitamin and mineral supplement. A similar approach in postmenopausal women already on HRT or Gynovite has been shown to raise progesterone levels approximately 50 per cent, and to improve their bone mineral density as well as their general well-being.

Only large studies that involve giving natural progesterone to post-menopausal women will answer the questions as to its effectiveness in controlling menopausal symptoms and bone loss. It is quite possible that a low progesterone level in a pre- or postmenopausal woman is a marker for a lack of robustness which in turn influences both long- and short-term health. A healthy diet and regular exercise with balanced nutrient levels seem to be simple ways in which to increase our robustness.

The WNAS has been helping women to overcome their menopausal symptoms for many years. To date we have not included progesterone as part of our programme. In view of the fact that our success rate is in the range of 90 per cent after four months' treatment, we reserve judgement on the progesterone issue until further medical research exists to support it.

Recent research carried out at King's College, University of London, showed that there is no scientific evidence to support the claims that natural progesterone is absorbed through the skin.

9

YOUR CONTINUED GOOD HEALTH

As you have seen, phytoestrogens have been shown to be a helpful tool when addressing the short-term symptoms of the menopause. When combined with an optimum nutritional intake, they have also been shown to play an important role in the prevention of a whole host of other conditions. These include heart disease, osteoporosis (the bone-thinning disease), as well as other oestrogen-dependent conditions, such as certain cancers, diabetes, dementia and even degenerative conditions, such as arthritis.

Sufficient research now suggests that the majority of women can sail through the menopause and beyond, maintaining a healthy heart and strong bones, without having to resort to HRT. This is just as well, as up to two-thirds of women who try HRT come off it within the first year due to side-effects or dissatisfaction and, as you have seen, there are specific groups of women who cannot take it for medical reasons.

HEART DISEASE

Let us look more closely at mechanisms to inhibit both heart disease and osteoporosis. Years ago, heart disease was a rarity, and probably associated with old age.

These days, in the Western world, heart disease has reached epidemic proportions. Although statistics in recent years are starting to decline in countries such as Australia, the USA and the UK, they are still rising in Eastern Europe. The situation has become so dire that the beginning of atherosclerosis (furring of the arteries) can sometimes even be detected in children. During the Korean war, researchers performed autopsies on nearly two thousand American soldiers in order to study war wounds. They found more than they bargained for, as they discovered that three-quarters of these young men, with an average age of 22, were already showing signs of the initial stages of atherosclerosis. Women over the age of 50, post-menopause, generally suffer more from high blood pressure and heart disease than men, which is thought to be attributable to the fact that they are no longer protected by natural oestrogen.

Whilst this may sound very depressing, consider the fact that whilst those living in the Western world are falling like flies, the majority of Asian communities generally reach old age with healthy blood vessels. We need to examine why this is so, and we don't need to look very far. During World War II, when food was rationed, there was a lack of meat and dairy products. Diets were largely based on vegetarian products such as grains, vegetables and beans, which meant that the consumption of animal fat was low. During this time, it just so happened that there was a dramatic decrease in heart disease.

Almost a hundred years ago it was discovered that animal protein, including meat, dairy products and eggs could induce atherosclerosis. In 1990 researchers at the University of California confirmed that diet can be as effective at combating atherosclerosis as either drugs or surgery. The research team devised a very low-fat vegetarian diet, exercise and meditation programme for a group of individuals with severely blocked arteries, which resulted in the arteries being cleared of plaque. Other fats, such as oleic acid found in olive oil and rapeseed oil, and polyunsaturated fatty acids derived from a variety of plants, fish oils and cold pressed linseed oil, have the reverse effect. They actually shift the balance towards the good High-Density Lipoprotein cholesterol (HDL). The degree of protection that these 'healthy oils' provided is debated, and of interest not only to the general public and doctors, but also to farmers and politicians. The majority of experts in Western countries recognise a need for the 'average' consumer to reduce their total fat intake by cutting down on saturated animal fats, maintaining a modest intake of polyunsaturates and making little change to the intake of oleic acid. No doubt the debate will continue for some time to come.

Many of the known risk factors also influence the balance between HDL and Low-Density Lipoprotein (LDL), the 'bad' cholesterol. For example, giving up smoking, correction of obesity and regular physical exercise may have a marked effect, reducing the total cholesterol and raising the ratio of good HDL to bad LDL. Doctors have not found it easy to raise HDL levels as they are largely determined by genetics. However, this is where soy and other phytoestrogens enter the picture.

" Alice's Story "

Alice is a 48-year-old wife, mother and grandmother, and works part-time as a dental nurse. She approached the WNAS in January 1999 after reading the first edition of this book, *Beat the Menopause Without HRT*, realising there were natural alternatives to help her through the menopause.

'The doctor prescribed HRT, and fortunately I experienced no side-effects, but I still suffered severely with irritability, loss of confidence and fatigue, and I also experienced uncomfortable breast tenderness and weight gain. I also have high blood pressure for which I take medication, but I would like to control it by natural means. When I read Maryon Stewart's Beat the Menopause Without HRT, I realised that I could help myself by making dietary modifications and taking nutritional supplements. The book was an excellent start, but I decided to seek more help so I phoned the advisory service and arranged a telephone consultation with the nurse.

I was asked to complete a comprehensive health questionnaire which detailed all my symptoms, both menopausal and general. I also had to record exactly what I ate and drank for one week. I returned my forms to the WNAS and someone contacted me by return to book an appointment. I had a telephone consultation with the WNAS and was advised to cut out all wheat and bran, which I was told can exacerbate hot flushes; reduce my tea and coffee consumption and start eating phytoestrogens (naturally occurring plant oestrogens). I made some simple dietary changes, substituting soya milk for cow's milk to provide me with a good serving of phytoestrogens, and replaced my much loved cup of tea with an amazing tea lookalike called Redbush. I must admit, I was concerned at the thought of cutting out wheat, but I now enjoy eating rye crispbreads and rice cakes and the WNAS provided me with a selection of tried and tested wheat-free cake and biscuit recipes!

I took nutritional supplements as well and by the time I had my second consultation, my symptoms had already started to lessen. The main things I noticed were fewer aches and pains, increased energy and I generally felt more mentally alert! I couldn't believe that cutting the wheat out could make me feel so much better and now, every time I eat it, my irritability is unbearable. I couldn't believe the rapid change, which made me even more inspired to get through the next few weeks.

After five months I had completed the course of treatment and all my symptoms were virtually non-existent. A bonus for me was that I had lost a stone *in weight and my blood pressure had dropped! All I can say is, contacting the WNAS for help was the best thing I have done for years – many thanks for your help.'*

The role of phytoestrogens in heart disease

It was discovered that soy protein lowers cholesterol levels almost by accident. In the late 1960s researchers set out to find out whether soy could be a palatable alternative protein to meat, and in doing so they noticed a marked reduction in cholesterol levels in the soya consumers. Almost a decade later, soy was again put under the microscope by Dr Sirtori at the University of Milan. He discovered that soy protein lowered cholesterol levels by an average of 14 per cent within two weeks, and by 21 per cent at the end of the three weeks. Since that time, much more research has been undertaken to look at the effects of soy on cholesterol levels. An analysis of 40 published studies was undertaken by Dr Kenneth Carrol at the University of Western Ontario. His conclusion was that 34 of the studies did produce a drop in LDL (bad cholesterol levels) in particular, by 15 per cent or more. Other more recent studies have shown that as well as reducing the level of LDL, soy has been successful in raising levels of HDL (the desirable cholesterol). Even genetically raised cholesterol levels have been seen to drop by 26 per cent in a four-week Italian study, published in 1991.

Another interesting study, conducted by Dr John Eden from Sydney, Australia, showed that menopausal women on Novogen Red Clover supplements, containing 40 mg of isoflavones per tablet, showed on average, an 18 per cent increase in the good cholesterol.

A recent study by Professor Kenneth Setchell, reported at the Third International Symposium on the *Role of Soy in Preventing and Treating Chronic Disease* in Washington DC, confirmed that it is possible to raise HDL whilst lowering LDL. His 12-week study, on 43 post-menopausal women consuming a soy-rich diet, containing 60–70 mg of total isoflavones each day, also highlighted the antioxidant effects of soy.

The benefits of phytoestrogens on lowering cholesterol levels and improving heart health are an extremely important breakthrough in medicine for post-menopausal women, who are no longer protected by oestrogen.

Furthermore, on 20th October 1999, the US Food and Drug Administration (FDA) approved a health claim for soy protein and its role in reducing the risk of coronary heart disease. This effectively means that food products that contain a minimum of 6.25 grams of soy protein per serving will be allowed to state on the label that in conjunction with a low-fat, low-cholesterol diet, the product may reduce the risk of heart disease. The health claim was developed by the FDA, which concluded, based on scientific evidence from more than 50 independent studies, that 25 grams of soy protein included in a daily diet that is low in saturated fat and cholesterol, reduces the risk of coronary heart disease.

The Italians are so convinced about the value of soy in lowering cholesterol that it is now provided free of charge by the Italian National Health Service to those with high cholesterol levels.

OSTEOPOROSIS

During our lives, there is a constant turnover of bone. Until we reach the age of approximately 35, we lose as much old bone each year as we make new, hence keeping the scales in balance. From then on we tend to lose about one per cent of our bone mass each year until we reach the menopause, at which point bone loss accelerates with a further loss of two or three per cent per year for up to 10 years.

In addition to the imbalance that develops between bone loss and the rate at which new bone is deposited, in osteoporosis there is also a reduction in both the amount of connective tissue and the mineral content of the bone. The loss of bone mass reduces its strength and increases the likelihood that the bone will break when pressure is brought to bear on it.

As a result of osteoporosis, one in three women and one in 12 men will suffer fractures of the hip, spine or wrist. Apart from the obvious pain and disability, osteoporosis often brings with it a loss of height and curvature of the spine, known in the UK as 'dowager's hump'. Within six months of sustaining a hip fracture, it is estimated that some 20 per cent of patients will die. However, what is not widely appreciated is that osteoporosis is both preventable and treatable.

Risk factors for osteoporosis

One of the functions of oestrogen is to help to keep our bone mass at an optimum level. As our oestrogen levels automatically fall, we become more susceptible to bone-thinning. However, oestrogen is not the only factor in determining bone strength and our chances of developing a fracture in later life.

Are you at risk?

Have you ever had, suffered from, or indulged excessively in any of the following:

- Poor diet, low in calcium, especially dairy products
- An early menopause, spontaneous or following surgery
- Thyroid or other hormonal problems
- Low body weight, or anorexia
- Petite build
- Cigarette smoking
- Regular and excessive alcohol consumption
- Lack of exercise and sedentary lifestyle
- Excessive physical activity, as in athletes or ballet dancers
- Steroid drugs
- Strong family history of osteoporosis
- Chronic illnesses affecting digestion, kidney and liver function.

Bone density

A number of dietary, lifestyle and environmental factors influence the strength and density of our bones throughout our lives. The mineral content of a woman's bones at the time of the menopause is not so much influenced by her current dietary intake, but by her past intake of calcium over the previous 40 or 50 years.

What determines the strength of our bones?

- Our diet, especially our intake of naturally occurring plant oestrogens and calcium during the growing years
- Physical activity, particularly weight-bearing exercise
- Hormonal factors, particularly the balance of oestrogen
- Genetic factors which determine the size of our bones and muscles.

The current standard diet in the UK is a factor in determining whether or not we develop osteoporosis in the same way as it is in determining the development of heart disease and cancer. Many of us consume a diet which, though adequate in the short term, does not provide a good or optimum intake of nutrients in the longer term, thus predisposing us to diseases such as osteoporosis.

Why is oestrogen so important?

Oestrogen maintains bone mass and helps with the constant process of bone remodelling. When oestrogen levels are optimum, our bones are constantly regenerating but when levels fall, calcium is no longer directed to our bones and the net result is bone loss.

Women who experience an early menopause, or who stop menstruating because of excessive dieting or exercise, will have depressed levels of oestrogen and as a result will be at greater risk of osteoporosis.

The role of phytoestrogens

Consuming a diet rich in plant foods will provide you with dozens of different types of phytochemicals that possess health-protective benefits. Apart from soy products and linseeds, which are rich sources of phytoestrogens, nuts, whole-grains, fruits and vegetables contain similar compounds and natural antioxidants.

What conventional treatments have to offer

Calcium
Calcium is particularly important. Average intakes in the UK, for women, are around 700 mg per day, the amount provided by just over a pint of milk. Some experts recommend daily intakes of 1000 mg or more of calcium, which is only achieved by a modest percentage of the UK population.

Vitamin D
Vitamin D is mainly derived from the action of sunlight on our skin and only small amounts come from the diet. It is needed to enhance the absorption of calcium from the diet.

Essential Fatty Acids
Recent research suggests that the essential fatty acids (EFAs) which are part of a healthy diet, also influence the balance of calcium in our bones. There are two types of essential fatty acids, the omega 3 series and the omega 6 series: the omega 3 series are derived from fish oils, oily fish including mackerel, herring, salmon, pilchards and sardines, as well as from some cooking oils such as rapeseed, linseed, soybean and walnuts.

The omega 6 series of EFAs are found in sunflower and corn oil – and margarine made from them, almonds and other nuts and seeds. These help to maintain healthy skin and also reduce the risk of heart disease. They also seem to help in the absorption of calcium from the diet.

The calcium controversy

Until recently, calcium intake was thought to be one of the most important factors in the prevention of osteoporosis. As we have said, average intakes in the UK, for women, are around 700 mg per day, whereas recommended daily intake is at least 1000 mg per day. However, many consume less than this, and doing so during childhood and early adult life will mean that they reach middle and old age with a low bone mass and a high risk of osteoporosis.

When you examine the international statistics for osteoporosis, a contradiction becomes apparent, for some of the nations with the highest calcium intake also have the highest rates of osteoporosis. Conversely, those with low intakes of calcium have some of the lowest rates of osteoporosis. What confuses the issue even further is that, according to anthropologists, over 10,000 years ago, only infants were able to drink milk, for we lacked the enzyme required to digest lactose (milk sugar). Hence, we open the door to an alternative underlying reason for the ever-escalating number of osteoporosis sufferers.

Half as many Japanese women suffer from hip fractures as women in the West, and women in countries such as Hong Kong and Singapore suffer fewer fractures still. One explanation could be that Asian women are more active. Japanese women, who traditionally sit on the floor, will probably have stonger muscles and bones as a result of their regular movements, compared with a woman leading a sedentary lifestyle. But there is more to it than that, as new research is beginning to unveil.

It has been established that animal protein promotes calcium loss but, on the positive side, it seems that soy protein has a protective effect. Animal studies have been conducted to compare the effect on bone health of Premarin (a hormone replacement made from pregnant mares' urine) and genistein. The result showed that low-dose genistein was able to prevent bone loss almost as well as Premarin. Dr John Anderson, at the University of North Carolina, who initiated the animal work, speculates that genistein's possible effects on bone may be due to its weak oestrogenic properties. Bone cells, like reproductive cells, have oestrogen receptor sites. At the time of the menopause, when oestrogen levels fall, the receptor sites in bone become redundant. It is likely that phytoestrogens continue the function of the natural oestrogen that was circulating around the body prior to the menopause, thus minimising bone loss.

Daidzein, another soy isoflavone, also seems to be providing us with good news on the bone front. A drug called Ipriflavone, which is made from daidzein, has been approved in Europe and Japan for the treatment of osteoporosis as it slows bone loss and stimulates the growth of new bone. Many positive studies of Ipriflavone on humans have been conducted. Overall, the studies seem to show that it effectively helps to improve bone density at a dose of 600 mg per day combined with 1000 mg of calcium. In the UK it is now being marketed as an over-the-counter supplement distributed by Solgar, and is available in most health-food shops.

Researchers are still trying to fathom out why soy seems to be calcium sparing when compared with animal protein. One theory is that soy protein has low levels of the sulphur containing amino acids, which cause the production of sulphate in the urine. Sulphate is known to work with the kidneys to prevent calcium from being reabsorbed into the bloodstream, and instead excreted through the urine. In addition to this, most high-protein foods contain phosphorus which, although it reduces the amount of calcium lost in the urine, it increases the calcium loss in our bowel motions. This may put regular meat eaters at an even greater disadvantage, as anyway meat contains low levels of calcium.

A study conducted by Professor Kenneth Setchell on 43 post-menopausal women consuming 60–70 mg of isoflavones per day for 12 weeks, found that the activity of the bone-dissolving cells decreased significantly by 13.9 per cent and the activity of the bone-forming cells also increased significantly by 10.2 per cent. These findings indicate reduced bone turnover with an isoflavone-rich diet. Another interesting study by Lee Alekel showed that 80 mg of isoflavone-rich isolated soy protein per day, for 24 weeks, was significantly bone sparing in the lumbar spine of perimenopausal women.

Another type of isoflavone, formononetin, has also recently been shown to help with bone regeneration. A six-month study, including 50 women, found a four per cent increase in bone regeneration of the cortical bone (involved in hip fractures) using Rimostil, which contains 50 mg of formononetin. This rate of increase is much more than that usually seen with oestrogen drugs, which also have little or no effect on cortical bone. This supplement is not available in the marketplace as yet, but will undoubtedly be a useful addition on the shelves in the not-too-distant future.

The way forward

The optimum regime for better bone health has to encompass all aspects of the research. We should of course be including calcium in the diet, but at the same time reducing our intake of animal protein, whilst increasing our consumption of soy protein. It appears the calcium-only crusade may have backed the wrong horse by treating osteoporosis as a deficiency disease. If it is a deficiency, it must be of oestrogen, rather than calcium.

How can we regenerate lost bone?

- By eating a healthy, well balanced diet, rich in essential nutrients, especially calcium, and the essential fatty acids
- By eating a phytoestrogen-rich diet
- By taking regular exercise, preferably weight-bearing (see the exercise chapter on page 165).

The value of exercise

At the time of the menopause, when we are most at risk of bone loss, exercise becomes a vital part of our schedule, and not just a nice idea. Research has shown that weight-bearing exercise (anything that involves putting weight through your bones) helps to stimulate the regeneration of bone tissue by reducing calcium loss. Plenty of exercise in childhood, including sport at school, helps to build up a high peak bone mass.

The consensus from studies is that you need to exercise moderately three or four times each week, for between 30 to 45 minutes each time, so long as you do not suffer with cardiovascular disease. For details about how to formulate your optimum exercise programme, refer to Chapter 13.

MIDLIFE MAYHEM

Despite the fact that phytoestrogens clearly play an important role in controlling the symptoms of the menopause, as well as helping to prevent other serious conditions, one could be forgiven for thinking that this was an official secret. Our survey of a thousand *Best Magazine* readers revealed that 83 per cent had never heard of phytoestrogens and many of those who had were not really sure what they were. Only 18 per cent of the sample thought that soy products would be helpful in preventing osteoporosis, and less than 15 per cent thought they would be helpful in preventing cancer, heart disease or high blood pressure. The results from the WNAS survey carried out on a thousand GPs were quite unexpected! It was amazing to see that as many as 17 per cent of doctors were recommending a soya rich diet, 18 per cent advised taking a phytoestrogen rich diet, which compared favourably with prescribing vitamin supplements and referral for psychotherapy, recommended by only 8 per cent of doctors. You can read more about this survey in Chapter 8 – The Phytoestrogen Factor.

On the plus side, and music to my ears, a massive 93 percent of the Best Survey participants said that they would be willing to modify their diet in order to improve their health prospects. Presumably, the fact that you are currently reading this book means that you are one of the 93 per cent. By following the instructions in Parts Three and Four of this book, you will have every opportunity to take advantage of all the non-drug, scientifically based, self-help measures that effectively help to overcome symptoms of the menopause, and preserve your health in the long term.

FINDINGS OF THE
WNAS OSTEOPOROSIS SURVEY

We carried out an Osteoporosis Survey in conjunction with Sanitarium, featured in the March 1999 edition of *Woman and Home* magazine. The survey was designed to determine whether or not there is a link between diet, lifestyle and osteoporosis. The average age of the respondents was 55.3 years and the range varied from 18 to over 80 years.

The survey shows that there is also much confusion about the actual nutritional and dietary requirements for the prevention of osteoporosis in terms of the optimum calcium intake and the types and quantities of food needed each week in order to maintain healthy bones. Just under three-quarters of the sample were unaware that soy products should be incorporated into an optimum diet to prevent osteoporosis and over half of the sample were not fully aware of the importance of calcium intake in the form of dairy products. In addition, nearly two-thirds of the sample are currently doing inadequate exercise to maintain their bone health.

- 5.2% of the sample were considered to be underweight – weighed less than 8 stones
- As many as 36.4% had at some time smoked, but only 4.4% were still smokers
- 30.9% of the sample said that they had a sedentary lifestyle
- Only 25% of the sample did three to four sessions of weight-bearing exercise per week. 15.8% did five to six sessions and 11% did seven or more
- 9.7% of the sample had experienced one or more fractures
- A staggering 25.6% had a relative with osteoporosis
- In reply to the question, 'Are you afraid of osteoporosis?' the response from the whole sample revealed that 27.2% were considerably afraid, 53.7% moderately and 14.2% were not afraid at all
- On average 50% of respondents felt that they should consume milk every day
- 11.5% felt that it was not essential to consume milk at all in order to prevent osteoporosis
- 74% of respondents felt that soy milk and soy products were *not* important in the prevention of osteoporosis.

A more detailed account of how to prevent the diseases and conditions associated with the ageing process can be found in my book *The Phyto Factor* (see page 321 for details).

PART THREE

THE NITTY GRITTY ON THE NATURAL APPROACH

10

DINING AT THE CAPTAIN'S TABLE – YOUR GUIDE TO A PHYTOESTROGEN-RICH DIET

Research so far does tell us about many of the foods that contain phytoestrogens. They are typically found in many common plant foods, including soy products, particularly soy milk, tofu and soy flour, plus organic linseeds – sometimes known as flaxseeds, lentils, chick peas, mung beans, sunflower, pumpkin and sesame seeds, many other beans, green and yellow vegetables, and the plant Red Clover. The following chart outlines the key phytoestrogen-rich foods and the quantity of the common forms of phytoestrogens per serving.

You will find a more extensive list of phytoestrogen-rich foods, and more than a hundred phytoestrogen-rich recipes in my book *The Phyto Factor* (see page 321). There are also some phytoestrogen-rich recipes and menus in the recipe section of this book.

Published research, as well as our own experience, points to the fact that a daily intake of phytoestrogens is necessary, preferably in split doses. In other words, little and often, as these compounds leave the body fairly rapidly. It is thought that isoflavones reach a peak in our blood within approximately six to eight hours. We have certainly found that by consuming a phytoestrogen-rich breakfast, perhaps the phyto muesli on page 296, together with So Good soy milk, and having a couple of additional 'phyto fixes' in the afternoon and evening, we can substantially increase the rate at which we can control menopausal hot flushes.

Along with the vast majority of key experts on phytoestrogens, I had the good fortune to attend the Third International Symposium on the Role of Soy in Preventing and Treating Chronic Disease, in Washington, USA. Whilst many researchers presenting new data at the Symposium currently feel that a diet rich in isoflavones is only likely to decrease hot flushes by 30 per cent, our experience is that, when combined with other aspects of the WNAS menopause programme, it is a valuable part of a highly effective, natural alternative to HRT, which aids the control of hot flushes in a relatively short time period.

HOW DOES THIS AFFECT THE DAILY DIET?

There is no need to be put off by the prospect of introducing phyto-estrogen-rich foods into your diet. There are so many different varieties that you will certainly find at least some of them enjoyable. It is not necessary to make radical changes to your diet unless you really want to.

You can simply get your daily phytoestrogen intake by combining So Good soy milk with fruit in the blender to make delicious fruit shakes, or blend silken tofu with fruit to make fruit whips. Additionally, there are savoury dips you can make that can be devoured with fresh veg-etable crudités and corn chips, or you can sample a slice of our phyto fruit loaf for tea.

If you are aiming to overcome severe and debilitating symptoms at the time of the menopause it is likely, in our experience, that you will need to consume at least 100 mg of isoflavones per day initially, com-bined with other important aspects of the WNAS programme, detailed in Part Four. This will enable you to emulate the Japanese consumption of daily phytoestrogens, but in a Western way.

THE MAIN TYPES OF PHYTOESTROGENS

Genistein is the most extensively studied isoflavone to date and, although it was identified as a plant oestrogen in 1966, it was not until 20 years later that its anti-cancer properties were recognised by medical scientists. Japanese researchers first discovered that genistein, found in soy products, was capable of blocking the signal that triggers the growth of a cancer cell, and that it was also able to inhibit the growth of a can-cerous tumour.

Daidzein the second major phytoestrogen to be discovered, like genis-tein acts as both an anti-cancer agent and an antioxidant. It also has a role to play in the prevention of bone mass depletion and, once again, is able to make cancer cells revert to normal.

Formononetin and Biochanin are two more oestrogenic isoflavones, which, although not present in soy, are chiefly derived from Red Clover, chickpeas, lentils and mung beans. Formononetin is a methy-lated daidzein, and biochanin is a methylated genistein. Their unique effects on human physiology are not possessed by the non-methylated isoflavones genistein and daidzein found in soy. As well as being cancer-protective compounds, they are also responsible for the positive lipid (blood fat)-lowering properties associated with traditional diets. *Lignans*, like soy products, possess both weak oestrogenic and anti-oestrogenic qualities, and are structurally similar to oestradiol, a form of oestrogen. Lignans are found in seeds, fruits and vegetables, with high amounts in linseeds, and are converted in humans by intestinal bacteria to hormone-like compounds. When linseeds are consumed, intestinal bacterial action results in the production of up to eight hundred times more of these lignans than from any other food.

HOW DO PHYTOESTROGENS WORK?

It seems that they are able to mimic and compete against oestrogen within the body as well as the potentially harmful environmental oestrogens (xenoestrogens), for the receptor sites at the entrance to the cells. So, for example, genistein, the look-alike oestrogen, is able successfully to occupy breast tissue, thus preventing the more potent natural oestrogen, produced by the body, from 'converting' normal cells into cancer cells. Because genistein is able to block the uptake of oestrogen, it acts as an 'anti-oestrogen', in a similar way to the drug tamoxifen administered to breast-cancer victims and, it would appear, without the side-effects.

THE PRINCIPLES OF A PHYTOESTROGEN-RICH DIET

Consuming a diet rich in plant foods will provide you with dozens of different types of phytochemicals that possess health-protective benefits. Apart from soy products and linseeds, nuts, whole-grains, fruits and vegetables contain an abundance of phenolic compounds, terpenoids, pigments and other natural antioxidants.

Milk

Like dairy milk, soy milk is a versatile liquid that can be consumed as a drink, or used in place of dairy milk in shakes, sauces, soups, cereals or in cooking. Until recently, drinks based on the soy bean have not proved popular with Westerners because of the unacceptable 'beany'

Foods rich in Isoflavones (mg/100 g)

Food	Isoflavones (mg/100 g)	Daidzein (mean)	Genistein (mean)	Reference
So Good soy beverage	25	5	16	Sanitarium NB: Also contains Glycitein (4 mg)
Provomel soy drinks and desserts	12	N/A	N/A	Provamel
Soy beans (mature, cooked, boiled without salt)	54.66	26.95	27.71	USDA*
Soy beans, mature seeds, sprouted, raw	40.71	19.1	21.6	USDA*
Soy beans, flakes (defatted)	125.82	36.97	85.69	USDA*
Soy bean paste	31.52	15.03	15.21	USDA*
Soy flour (defatted)	131.9	57.47	71.21	USDA*
Silken tofu (Vitasoy soft)	29.24	8.59	20.65	USDA*
Tofu (firm, prepared with calcium sulphate and nigari)	24.74	9.44	13.35	USDA*
Tofu (raw, ordinary, prepared with calcium sulphate)	23.61	9.02	13.6	USDA*
TVP (Textured Vegetable Protein)	22.9	7.9	11.8	Tham et al, 1998
Tempeh, cooked	53.0	19.25	31.55	USDA*
Tempeh burger	29.0	6.4	19.6	USDA*
Miso	42.55	16.13	24.56	USDA*
Miso soup mix, dry	60.39	24.93	35.46	USDA*
Soy protein isolate	97.43	33.59	59.62	USDA*
Soy cheese, unspecified	31.32	11.24	20.08	USDA*
Soy noodles, flat	8.5	0.9	3.7	USDA*
Soy & linseed bread (Vogel's)	37.9	N/A	N/A	Stevens & Co Australia
*Prevacan cereal bar (soy and flaxseed)	33.6 mg per bar	12.8 mg per bar	17.6 mg per bar	Phytogenics Limited

[*Inconclusive at time of going to press]

* USDA-Iowa State University Database on the Isoflavone Content of Foods (1999). Website address: www.nal.usda.gov/fnic/foodcomp/Data/isoflav/isoflav.html
N/A = Figures not available

Foods rich in Lignans (mg/100 g)

Food	Lignans	Reference
Linseeds (flaxseeds)	371	Mazur 1998
Linseeds (flaxseeds)	59 mg per tablespoon	Mazur 1998
Pumpkins seeds	21.37	Adlercreutz & Mazur 1997
Bramble	3.74	Mazur 1998
Strawberry	1.58	Mazur 1998
Lingonberry	1.51	Mazur 1998
Cranberry	1.054	Mazur 1998
Otaheite gooseberry	3.05	Mazur 1998
Prevacan bar	3 mg per bar	Phytogenics Ltd
Chinese green tea	3.085	Mazur 1998
Prince of Wales black tea	2.725	Mazur 1998
Earl Grey black tea	1.787	Adlercreutz & Mazur 1997
Chinese black tea	1.14	Mazur 1998

Foods rich in Coumestans, Formononetin and Biochanin A (mg/100 g)

Food	Coumestrol	Formononetin	Biochanin A	Reference
Red clover		13220	8330	USDA*
Alfalfa sprouts	0	261	0	USDA*
Alfalfa sprouts mixed with clover sprouts	466	1771	2946	USDA*
Soy sprouts	38.6	0		USDA*
Clover sprouts	28.1	2.28	0.44	USDA*
Chinese peas, cooked	0	0	9.31	USDA*
Split peas, round	8.11	0	0	USDA*
Pinto beans, dry	3.61	Trace	0.56	USDA*
Garbanzo beans, dry	0	0.14	1.78	USDA*
Black-eyed beans, dry	0	0	1.73	USDA*
Pink beans, dry	0	1.05	0	USDA*
Mung beans, dry	0	0.61	0	USDA*
Split peas, yellow and green	0	0	0.86	USDA*

* USDA-Iowa State University Database on the Isoflavone Content of Foods (1999).
Website address: www.nal.usda.gov/fnic/foodcomp/data/isoflav/isoflav.html

taste. Milk, made by the traditional whole-bean method, can sometimes cause wind and bloating as it is more difficult to digest. SGI, the makers of So Good, has overcome this problem by using a soy protein and combining it with vegetable oil, maltodexrin, sugar, vitamins and minerals, to produce a dairy milk lookalike. It is lactose-free and has therefore been used by those intolerant to lactose and by vegans. Although it does not contain as much vitamin D, calcium or vitamin B12 as dairy milk, So Good is fortified with these. As well as being sold as plain milk, flavoured varieties are often available, including chocolate, strawberry, mocha and vanilla, although these may have a lower isoflavone content than the plain milk. Also available are low-fat varieties, such as So Good Lite, Granose reduced fat, Plamil Lite and own-brand products.

Linseeds

Linseeds are a rich source of omega-3 fatty acids which are predominantly derived from oily fish. These fatty acids are essential for a healthy nervous system, soft skin, bright eyes, a strong immune system ... the health benefits are immense. Fresh organic golden linseeds (Linusit Gold are much nicer than brown seeds) can be combined with breakfast cereal each day. Two tablespoons of seeds, either whole or, preferably, ground, should be sprinkled over the cereal or used in the muesli as an ingredient.

Linusit Gold can be ground either in a coffee grinder or a blender, or with a pestle and mortar, and then stored in a sealed container in the refrigerator. They can also be sprinkled over salads, fruit salads, cakes, combined with yogurt or milk, and even included when baking fresh bread. It is important to consume plenty of liquid with linseeds so, if you are not combining them with milk, juice or yogurt, have a drink afterwards.

11

THE VALUE OF ISOFLAVONE-RICH SUPPLEMENTS

As only a relatively small percentage of menopausal women continue with Hormone Replacement Therapy in the long-term, the 'menopause market' is probably perceived as a goldmine by the manufacturers of non-drug products. In the USA, an estimated 30 million menopausal women do **not** take HRT, four per cent take it in Italy, whilst in the UK 15–20 per cent of all menopausal women take it (source: Amarant Trust, UK). Australian surveys show that approximately 30–40% of menopausal women are currently undergoing HRT. You don't have to be a mathematician to work out that this means that currently there are millions of women worldwide who may be looking for a solution to their menopause symptoms, usually independently of their doctors.

The last few years have seen an abundance of mainly soy-based supplements coming onto the market. Sadly, the vast majority of these are not scientifically based and, according to research, will not necessarily protect us in the same way as soy-based foods. In fact, eminent professors, including Professor Kenneth Setchell and Professor Herman Adlercreutz, are actively dissuading us from using soy-based supplements, until further research has been undertaken.

The Japanese traditionally consume soy products within their diet, in relatively small quantities, meaning that their isoflavone intake from soy is little and often. One of the dangers with soy-based supplements is that they administer a large amount of isoflavones in one dose. Additionally, studies have shown that they do not have the same effect as soy-based foods on symptoms of the menopause and heart disease prevention for example.

But despite these findings there is a real need for an isoflavone-rich supplement, for the majority of Western women are not likely to consume a similar diet to the Japanese. The WNAS menopause programme has successfully managed to disguise soy milk, flour and tofu within our recipes, which you will find in the menu and recipe section beginning on page 263. We aim to encourage women to consume many of the milligrams of daily phytoestrogens they require in the form of food. However, initially, when symptoms are severe and debilitating, we find great value in combining food intake with a supplement. The supplement we use delivers 40 mg of the four main isoflavones per tablet in the form of Red Clover, another isoflavone-rich substance, rather than soy. You will see from page 152 that the supplement of our choice is a scientifically based Red Clover preparation produced by the Sydney-based company, Novogen.

A recent US study has validated the effectiveness and safety of Novogen Red Clover. The study, conducted by Tufts University School of Medicine and New York University School of Medicine, showed that menopausal women who took a single tablet of Red Clover daily experienced a reduction in the intensity and number of hot flushes. Hot flushes were reduced by 56 per cent (from 8.1 per day to 3.6 per day) after eight weeks. Intensity of hot flushes also decreased by 56 per cent, and nightsweats decreased in intensity by 52%. Hot flushes and nightsweats are the two most common symptoms in menopausal women. The other good news was that Red Clover did not cause a thickening of the endometrial lining, which is a complication commonly associated with HRT. The women in the study also reported no side-effects or weight gain from taking Red Clover.

We have been using Novogen Red Clover as part of the WNAS menopause programme for the last two years. Within the first few months of experimenting with the product by giving samples to our patients to try, we discovered that the hot flushes and the nightsweats were being controlled much more quickly. Whereas it used to take us at least three or four months to control hot flushes, once we included the Red Clover supplement into the programme patients began returning for their follow-up appointment just one month after their initial consultation, delighted that both their flushes and nightsweats were far milder. This was excellent news for the WNAS team as well as the patients themselves.

The women included in the study had been suffering, on average, with their menopausal symptoms for almost four years, and their average age was 51. To control their symptoms, 37 of the women had previously tried HRT and half of them had experienced side-effects.

Results of the WNAS Menopause Programme incorporating Novogen Red Clover

Severe symptoms	Degree of improvement
Palpitations	95%
Insomnia	83%
Irritability	79%
Hot Flushes	77%
Loss of confidence	72%
Dry vagina	70%
Night sweats	60%
Loss of libido	60%
Panic attacks	55%

Novogen Red Clover is available from many chemists and health-food shops, and is also available from the WNAS mail order service. For details, see page 309.

« Gabrielle Battersby's Story »

'I suffered severely with hot flushes, to the point of having disturbed sleep most nights. I would wake up, throwing back the covers in an attempt to cool down, then find it very difficult getting back to sleep. My broken sleep pattern was having a negative effect on my concentration and social life. I approached the WNAS out of sheer desperation and they sent me a detailed questionnaire to complete, which asked me about my symptoms and diet. I returned the questionnaire and spoke to a nutritionist who gave me comprehensive dietary recommendations. I was told to cut out wheat and caffeine, which exacerbate hot flushes, and eat plenty of fresh fruit and vegetables and oily fish. By substituting soy milk for cow's milk, I would ensure a good intake of naturally occurring plant oestrogens (phytoestrogens) which alleviate menopausal symptoms. I was told to take Gynovite – a multi-vitamin/mineral formulated specifically for women going through the menopause, vitamin E and Panax Ginseng to alleviate the flushes. After only one week of following the dietary and supplement guidelines, I'd only had one disturbed night! Thanks to the WNAS I feel healthier, my hot flushes have drastically diminished and I have so much more energy.'

REDRESSING THE BALANCE

Through research over the years at the WNAS we have come to realise that the menopause is often the time when the nutritional cracks appear. A combination of years of wear and tear, pregnancy and breast-feeding, can challenge our nutrient stores, and the lack of knowledge about how to replace what time and nature have taken leave many women in a depleted state at the time of this important transition. Replacing the important nutrients, including magnesium, zinc, B vitamins and essential fatty acids, is vital for brain chemical metabolism as well as normal hormone function. In order to redress the balance as part of the WNAS menopause programme, for years we have been successfully using a magnesium-rich multi-vitamin and mineral supplement, Gynovite. This supplement was formulated by a professor of obstetrics and gynaecology, and designed for women at the time of the menopause and beyond. It has been shown positively to influence brain chemistry, hormone function and to help to improve our bone mass. Natural vitamin E has also been shown to be moderately helpful in controlling hot flushes.

Matching supplement to symptom

Problem	Type of supplement	Daily dosage	Available from
Hot flushes & nightsweats	Novogen Redclover	1 × 40 mg tablet	WNAS mail order
Osteoporosis	Novogen Redclover	1 × 40 mg tablet	WNAS mail order

Herbal supplements

- *Novogen Red Clover* This advanced phytoestrogen-rich supplement is a natural dietary isoflavone food supplement for women, delivering 40 mg of isoflavones per tablet, which allows us to top up on naturally occurring phytoestrogens. It is made from the herb Red Clover, containing high concentrations of the isoflavones genistein, daidzein, formononetin and biochanin. Red Clover is the richest source of these four oestrogenic isoflavones, having up to 10 times the levels of the next richest source, soy. Novogen Red Clover is the only scientifically based supplement on the market capable of delivering all the isoflavones in balanced proportions.

- *Panax Ginseng* This has been shown to be moderately helpful in controlling hot flushes, especially when used in conjunction with natural vitamin E. In fact, before we began using Novogen Red Clover, this was the combination of our choice. Ginseng is on the list of phytoesterols, the oestrogen-like substances. It comes in supplement form from health-food shops, and can also be used in the form of tea.
- *St John's Wort (hypericum)* This has been used in the treatment of depression for many years, and is thought to be more effective in the treatment of moderate depression, and to have fewer side-effects than conventional antidepressants. A 12-week German study of 111 women experiencing libido problems at the time of the menopause showed that 60 per cent of the women significantly regained their libido.

Other herbal supplements have been suggested to help to re-balance hormones. Some of the best known herbs are *dong quai* and *black cohosh*, both of which contain plant-like oestrogen substances, and may be worth a try. *Agnus castus*, another herb, has been shown to help with the treatment of headaches. These remedies are usually available from health-food shops.

12

COMPLEMENTARY THERAPIES AND THE MENOPAUSE

Holistic medicine looks at the whole person: the mind, the body and the spirit and how they interact. So, as well as dealing with symptoms on a nutritional level, it's important to make sure that you are functioning on an optimum level across the board. The years during which you may have suffered as a result of not eating the right diet, being pregnant and breast-feeding, coping with stressful situations and perhaps premenstrual symptoms before your menopause may well have taken their toll. The body is a complicated but delicate network of bones, muscles, ligaments, nerves, organs and blood vessels. Physical symptoms and nervous tension can affect the smooth running of the body processes. If your symptoms are intense, before and when you start your nutritional programme in Part Four, you might consider the value of acupuncture or acupressure, herbal medicine or cranial osteopathy as a means of speeding up the recovery process. They are powerful tools and can help to bring about the speedy relief of symptoms.

ACUPUNCTURE

Traditional Chinese medicine can be useful in the treatment of female health problems. According to the severity of the problem, there are two levels at which treatment can be taken. The first level is appropriate for severe symptoms and involves consulting an acupuncturist. Many of the problems mentioned, including hot flushes, insomnia, depression, aches and pains, mood swings and headaches may well respond to treatment by acupuncture. The second level involves acupressure (see page 156).

Chinese medicine is quite different from Western medicine in that it considers symptoms rather than named conditions and the diagnosis and subsequent treatment address the whole person – mind, body and lifestyle.

The principles

In order for good health to exist, Chinese medicine works on the premise that a universal energy known as *chi*, which has two complementary qualities known as *yin* and *yang*, must be in perfect balance. The term *yin* encompasses the feminine principle – cold and the state of rest – whereas *yang* includes the male principle – heat and activity. These principles are active in appropriate degrees in both men and women. When the balance is upset, illness results.

Chi flows through the 12 meridians or channels of the body, which are each associated with a particular organ, such as the lungs, liver or spleen. Herbal remedies and acupuncture are used to restore the balance of *yin* and *yang* and thus promote healing.

Treatment

As well as taking an in-depth medical history the Chinese doctor will take your pulse at six different points on each wrist to get the measure of each of the 12 vital organs of the body. Your tongue will also be inspected closely as its texture reflects the condition of the vital organs.

Acupuncture uses stainless-steel needles, which are inserted into specific points, or meridians, in order to affect the energy flowing to an organ. The needles, which remain in place for approximately 20 minutes, don't actually hurt: they may tingle and cause a mild ache or heat sensation.

You should always consult a properly trained and registered practitioner. You can usually obtain information from your public library or Citizens' Advice Bureau. A register is published by the Council for Acupuncture, listing all members of the five recognised and affiliated professional bodies.

Of the nine per cent of our midlife survey sample who tried acupuncture, 74 per cent found it helpful.

ACUPRESSURE OR SHIATSU

A second level of treatment, more appropriate to the minor or occasional problems that you can sometimes alleviate by self-assessment and home treatment, is *shiatsu*, the Japanese finger-pressure method, sometimes called acupressure. In this system, the body is influenced in various ways by the stimulation of key points, found along the course of energy channels circulating near the surface of the skin. These are the same as acupuncture meridians, but the points are stimulated by pressure rather than needles.

For *shiatsu* to be effective, it's important to apply the right kind of pressure for an appropriate length of time. It's no good pushing pressure points like 'magic buttons' and it's important to recognise by feel whether what you are doing is correct. Providing you adopt the right approach, *shiatsu* may be very helpful. You can enlist the help of a friend or perform it on yourself.

Shiatsu is particularly useful for treating musculo-skeletal problems, such as arthritis, stress, fatigue, and circulatory problems which are often exacerbated during the menopause.

Here is a summary of the method and a description of how to find just a few of the most useful points for some of the troubles mentioned.

Depression and anxiety

First, try working with repeated steady thumb pressure along your inner leg between the edge of the bone and the calf muscle. Also, there is a good point to press firmly two inches above your wrist, in between the tendons at the centre of your inner arm.

Breathing is very important to get your energy flowing smoothly, so try this simple exercise. Kneel on a cushion or carpet and join your hands together with your fingers back-to-back while pointing your fingertips towards your own upper abdomen. Let your relaxed fingers press into the centre, below the ribs but above the navel. As you do this, lean gently forward and exhale. The pressure should lend a little force to the exhalation. Wait for the inhalation to come naturally and raise yourself back again to the upright kneeling position while breathing in. Go gently at first, repeating the action with every breath, leaning a bit further on to your fingers each time. The abdominal muscles may seem tight or tender but try to relax fully at the end of each breath while leaning forward. Only do this 10 times. You may move your fingers up and down or a little way along your ribs to explore for any tension. Afterwards sit quietly for a minute. You may feel like having a good stretch before getting up.

Insomnia and headaches

Work with your fingertips along the base of your skull behind your head where it joins your neck. Feel for any sensitive hollows where your muscles meet the bony ridge and, leaning your head back, let your fingers penetrate. Hold for a few breaths. (If you do this for a friend, support her forehead with one hand and use your other hand to find points with finger and thumb on either side of her neck, pressing inward and upward.) For frontal headaches, lean forward. Let your fingertips support your forehead just below your eyebrows: it may feel tender, but breathe and relax for several seconds. Another useful point for headaches can be found by pressing hard into the fleshy area between your finger and thumb – press towards the edge of the bone on the forefinger side.

Also, work generally along the inside edges and soles of your feet, pressing especially around the inside ankle area.

Hot Flushes

The kidneys are the foundation of *yin* and *yang*, responsible for the stages of human development and decline. So it's important to support the kidneys and harmonise the kidneys and the heart. It's regarded a bit like fire and water and, as the water ebbs at the time of the menopause, the fire begins to flare up: hence the flushes.

As the menopause is considered to be an energetic disharmony of the kidney *chi*, there are two main areas that are worth working on to alleviate flushing and perspiration.

First, give pressure to points on the heart channel with your thumb held firmly at right angles. There are two or three points on the inside of your wrist, on the little-finger side along a line extending an inch or so up your arm from the wrist crease itself, which is just above the bone. Maintain the pressure for several seconds on each point, breathing and relaxing as you do it. Repeat this on your other wrist.

Then work points along the kidney channel on each foot. Following a line from approximately two inches above your inner ankle, press firmly – inching down between the bone and the Achilles' tendon on to your heel, on around and beneath your ankle bone and along the inside of your foot to the point in the middle of the sole, approximately one-third of the distance back from the toes. (If you look under the sole of your foot while you crunch up your toes, there is a little groove at this point.)

As the kidney is the target area, general massage and thumb or finger pressure around the kidney or the lower back is also useful. Plenty of rest and relaxation to regenerate the energy of the kidneys is also advisable.

If this approach really interests you, you could look for *shiatsu* classes in your area. If you do not know of any, write to the secretary of the Shiatsu Society whose address is listed in Appendix 4 at the back of the book. The Society will send you a list of qualified teachers.

HERBAL MEDICINE

Herbal medicine is older and more ubiquitous than any other type of medication on earth: everywhere which has been inhabited by people and plants has had its own herbal medicine. The great majority of plant medicines in use today were discovered by hunter-gatherers and so pre-date history itself. There is very good evidence that in all past and present hunter-gatherer societies, the responsibilities for gathering and learning about plant medicine belonged to women. So perhaps we can trust that, so far as the menopause is concerned, it was the afflicted who discovered their own remedies.

As civilisations emerged, men became involved with agriculture and medicine and tended to form analytical systems. As China, for example, evolved the polar principles of *yin* and *yang*, so European medicine relied on the concepts of *love* and *strife*: these resolved into the four elements which in turn were thought to be represented in the body by the four bodily fluids or *humours*. Many of these concepts still inform the best herbal medical practice in the West today, along with naturopathic ideas, many learned from native North Americans. Like Chinese medicine, European herbal medicine places great emphasis upon diet and exercise and other environmental factors.

The Principles

While herbal medicine aims to treat your current condition, it takes into consideration your past history from the time you were born, and the health of your parents at the time of conception. So, even if your symptoms are the same as your neighbour's, your prescriptions are unlikely to be the same. In other words, while we are all subject to the same biophysical laws, each of us has a unique tissue profile and therefore the treatment (by a once-living plant organism) needs to be unique.

When addressing symptoms of the menopause, the herbal specialist will treat the menstrual cycle: after all, the pituitary gland and the hypothalamus are still functioning, despite the falling levels in oestrogen. Their approach still respects the menstrual cycle, and the herbal remedies aim to reinstate cyclical behaviour. The herbalist wishes to support the adrenal axis and to redress target-organ sensitivity, because that contributes to the menopausal woman's difficulty with heat control. The aim is to enable the woman's body to convert heat into energy, mainly by treating her liver.

The treatment

The prescription you will receive may consist of a combination of a few or many different herbs. Sometimes you will be given herbs to take at different times of the day and, on occasion, herbs for different times of the month, depending on whether you are perimenopausal or post-menopausal. Some of the herbs used in prescriptions are well known, like *vitex agnus castus*, sage, vervain, St John's wort, mother wort, false unicorn root, hops and French marigold.

Although herbal medicine cannot claim to initiate bone regeneration – to my knowledge there have been no studies to demonstrate this – they have been shown to help speed up the healing of broken bones, and also to aid *absorption* of minerals from the digestive tract.

Of the 24 per cent of our midlife survey sample who tried herbs, 80 per cent found them useful.

If you wish to consult a trained herbalist, you will find the address to contact in Appendix 5.

HOMOEOPATHY

Samuel Hahnemann, the founder of homoeopathy, developed a system of treating sick people with safe medicine. The word homoeopathy comes from two Greek words: *omio* which means 'same' and *pathos* which means 'suffering'. Whereas allopathic medicine (the conventional medicine we know in the West) aims to treat symptoms with a drug that will produce an opposite effect, homoeopathy treats 'like with like'. A homoeopathic remedy is designed to produce the same symptoms as those you are suffering and in doing so aims to cancel them out. The dosages used are minute and may contain none of the original material. In this latter case, it is thought that the medicine, pill or liquid, contains an energy, or 'spirit', of the original medicine. Even these extreme dilutions have been shown to be effective in treating many conditions, including arthritis and hayfever. Many people appear to have benefited by their use, including women with menopausal symptoms.

The WNAS midlife survey revealed that of the 14 per cent who tried homoeopathy, 76 per cent found it helpful.

The principles

Homoeopathy is an approach to treatment which aims to assist Nature with her own process of healing rather than by-passing her altogether.

Like other holistic treatments it treats each person as an individual. A trained homoeopath takes an exceedingly thorough history before suggesting the most suitable remedy. It's very much a gentle preventive method of treatment which works best in conjunction with improved dietary and lifestyle measures.

Many people regularly use homoeopathic remedies to help themselves, for anything from coughs and colds to menstrual problems. While the British royal family continue to be staunch supporters of homoeopathy, it will undoubtedly remain an option for us all. The remedies are widely available, sometimes even on National Health prescriptions, and they are reasonably priced. Sometimes it's trial and error until you find the remedy that suits you, but it may well be worth persisting.

The treatment

Dr Andrew Lockie and Dr Nicola Geddes wrote an excellent reference book called *The Women's Guide to Homoeopathy*. Their view is that menopausal problems represent imbalances which have been present in your body for a long time. As well as recommending homoeopathic remedies, they also suggest that women should look at their diet, take exercise and correct any PMS symptoms as well as adopting a positive attitude and self-value before the onset of the menopause. There are specific remedies to fit symptom pictures and a trained homoeopath would be able to decide which remedy is most suited to your needs.

Sepia and sulphur are just two of the many remedies that may be indicated for hot flushes and nightsweats. There is also a wide choice of remedies for poor memory, depression, insomnia, anxiety attacks, irritability, headaches and confusion – in fact, the list is almost endless.

If you want to seek professional help, the addresses of The Faculty of Homoeopathy and The British Homoeopathic Association are in the Useful Addresses section in Appendix 5. If you are lucky, you may find a qualified medical homoeopath in your area or, better still, in a local NHS practice.

CRANIAL OSTEOPATHY

It's not uncommon, through the wear and tear of everyday life, for subtle back or neck problems to occur. I have seen many resistant, longstanding headaches cured by some good osteopathic manipulation. It is certainly worth having a check-up with a qualified osteopath or cranial osteopath if you feel tension building up in your back or neck or if you suffer from regular headaches.

The principles

Cranial osteopathy, or cranio-sacral therapy as it is known, is a specialised form of osteopathy and is gentle yet potent. The aim is gently to coax the muscles, tendons, joints and connective tissue to establish correct functions and release restrictions, thus restoring normal circulation, the flow of energy and glandular secretions.

The cranio-sacral mechanism is made up of the cranium (the skull), the sacrum (the bone at the base of the spine), the membranes surrounding the brain, the spinal cord and the fascia of continuous, clingfilm-like sheet that surrounds the muscles, organs, joints and bones. The tension of this fascia, the clingfilm-like lining, is all-important. If you have ever worn an all-in-one pants suit that is too tight or too short, you will have felt uncomfortable. If the tension in the body's fascia becomes too tight, you can't just take it off and it's possible that body functions can be affected in the long-term.

Cranial osteopathy works on two basic principles: first, that structure can affect function, and second, that impairment in the structure, or reduced mobility, will affect blood flow. Blood flow is of supreme importance in osteopathy and the treatment is aimed at improving local circulation and freeing-up the nerve supply.

Everything in the body moves with the cranial rhythm, which is the rhythm of the central nervous system. It's a movement like a breathing rhythm, which is constant, even when we sleep. The movement helps blood to flow generally and improves local circulation after trauma.

If there are restrictions to soft tissue, like muscles, to the fascia or to the membranes, then blood, lymph and cerebral spinal-fluid is restricted; as a result, nutrition to that area is affected.

The treatment

In the case of hormonal problems, circulation is regarded as being very important. The pituitary gland can be affected in several ways. For example, undue tensions or stresses in the membranes around the pituitary stalk affect the circulation and blood supply, which in turn results in a change of function.

The treatment for women suffering with menopausal symptoms is often aimed at improving pituitary function and balancing the function of the adrenal glands and the pelvis.

T'AI CHI

T'ai Chi is a Chinese movement therapy that was practised by Taoist monks in the 13th century, but its exact origins are difficult to trace. Derived from the words for 'great', 'ultimate' and 'fist', t'ai Chi can be translated as 'supreme ultimate power'. This therapy was suppressed during the Cultural Revolution (1966–69), but it has since been promoted by the Chinese government as a form of preventive health care. In the West it is now one of the most popular movement therapies of all ages. The key principles of t'ai Chi aim to ensure the smooth flow of 'life energy' through the body's meridians. It is recommended therapy for conditions of old age, improving vitality, enhancing mental and physical control and generally promoting optimum health.

Whichever holistic therapy you choose to explore, it's important to put yourself in the hands of a qualified practitioner. These days, all the recognised 'alternative' therapies have official associations which keep registers of qualified practitioners. It is best to check, as there are, sadly, many non-qualified people who are not to be recommended. You will find the addresses of all the relevant associations on the Useful Address list in Appendix 4.

THE HOLISTIC APPROACH
IN PRACTICE

From our *Woman's Realm* survey of 500 women we were able to get some insight into the kind of alternative therapies women have turned to, and the degree of success experienced. As you will see from the following chart, even more of the women on HRT had been using alternative therapies than those not on HRT. Seventy-five per cent of the non-HRT users had tried one or more therapy, compared with 80 per cent of those who had tried HRT. While the alternative therapies are perfectly compatible with HRT, I don't think that explains why more women who had previously tried HRT had also tried more alternative therapy. As over 67 per cent of our sample experienced side-effects with HRT, it's understandable that they then sought alternative help.

How Popular were the Alternative Therapies?

Therapy	240 Non-HRT Users	254 HRT Users	Benefit Non-HRT Users	Benefit HRT Users
Vitamin/Minerals	60%	57.5%	80%	74%
Diet therapy	42%	47%	74%	65%
Homoeopathy	10%	14.5%	62.5%	51.5%
Herbal remedies	12.5%	14%	60%	66%
Acupuncture	4%	5.5%	33%	36%
Yoga	9%	10%	68%	62%
Reflexology	4%	6%	40%	47%
Other	11%	7.5%	92%	68%

The only conclusions that we can draw from this is that a lot of women are trying a lot of therapies with some degree of success. In fairness, our survey was not detailed enough to find out specific details about therapies and whether women had a course of treatment or a one-off session. We know that making a few dietary changes may be nowhere near as effective as following a whole programme which has been tailor-made for you.

13

THE BENEFITS OF EXERCISE

Laura Topper holds a Master of Science degree in Exercise and Health Behaviour and specialises in physical activity and the menopause transition. In addition to continuing her research in this particular field, Laura is a lecturer and assessor and uses her wealth of knowledge to educate exercise providers on the benefits of physical activity throughout all life-stages.

I am delighted that she was able to contribute to *Cruising Through the Menopause* by writing this chapter.

PHYSICAL ACTIVITY AND MANAGEMENT
OF THE MENOPAUSE

At the turn of this century a woman's average lifespan was 50 years, and the major cause of mortality was cardiovascular heart disease (CHD). Now, on average, women will live one third of their lives after the menopause. These extra years that we now have are due to improvements in medication and an improved standard of living. However, we have also become less physically active.

Physical activity is now recognised as being a major contributor to improved health throughout all life stages. In fact, research shows that physical inactivity may be the prime risk factor for poor health – ahead of smoking, obesity, diabetes and a family history of cardiovascular heart disease. Furthermore, an active lifestyle has been found to improve health-related quality of life throughout both women's and men's lives.

It is acknowledged that women's bodies respond positively to physical activity. They benefit both physiologically and psychologically, so my aim in this chapter is to inform you of the health improvements that can be obtained through active living.

Physiologically there are, of course, many changes that may naturally occur during the menopause. Because of the falling oestrogen levels at this time, the body's ability to renew bone is reduced which may lead to an increased risk of fracture due to osteoporosis. Furthermore, an increase in low-density lipoproteins ('bad' cholesterol') and a decrease in high-density lipoproteins ('good' cholesterol) may collectively be responsible for factors such as excess body fat, the onset of diabetes and an increased risk of heart disease. During the menopause, oestrogen production from the ovaries is reduced to essentially nothing and the body has to rely on minimal amounts of oestrogen released from adrenal glands and fat stores. It is therefore usual during this time for these fat stores to increase in order to hold more oestrogen, and this may bring about unnecessary weight gain. However, proper nutrition and physical activity together can control weight.

Both osteoporosis and cardiovascular heart disease (CHD) have stirred up much interest in the fields of research and, more recently, it has been found that by adopting a physically active lifestyle during the menopause women may actually be reducing the risk of both of these conditions. Later on in this chapter I will be outlining exercise guidelines that are recommended by the American College of Sports Medicine (ACSM) for improving bone mineral density and cardiorespiratory fitness, but for now I would like to look further at the effects of physical activity on bone turnover and the health of the heart, as these areas are both vulnerable at the time of the menopause.

THE EFFECTS OF PHYSICAL ACTIVITY ON BONE DENSITY

Osteoporosis is defined as a disease which is characterised by low bone mass and deterioration of bone tissue which leads to bone fragility and the consequent increase in fracture risk. Of course, as outlined in Chapter 9, many factors come into play in relation to risk factors and low bone density, but my focus is on the effects of physical activity on bone turnover. There does not yet appear to be evidence to show that physical activity can actually prevent osteoporosis; however, many studies have found that significant associations exist between physical activity and increased bone mass in postmenopausal women. Knowing that we are able to improve bone status is extremely encouraging. One common predictor for bone mass density (BMD) during the menopausal years is whether peak bone mass was reached during earlier life (up to the late 20s). Of course, this information is often unknown as it is unlikely that a bone density scan would have been performed during our teens and 20s. However, identifying our activity levels during these earlier years may give a very rough guide to levels of peak bone mass.

In order to improve BMD as well as following the dietary recommendations suggested, weight-bearing activities are important. As you may recall from Chapter 9, until we reach our peak bone mass, new bone cells are laid down (bone formation) in abundance and old bone cells die (bone resorption) at a slower rate. However, after we have reached peak bone mass, this process reverses itself which means that the old cells die more rapidly and bone formation slows down.

Whilst participating in weight-bearing activities, an electrical charge is stimulated that encourages a transaction between muscle and bone to promote calcium deposition from the blood to the bone, promoting bone formation. In addition to this, in premenopausal women there may be a significant relationship between increased muscle strength and greater BMD.

One further point that must be addressed here is fracture due to falling, particularly for women in the menopause transition and beyond who may have low BMD and osteoporosis. The psychological effects of a fall may be highly devastating and, in many cases, the recovery from a fracture due to a fall may be traumatic. Strong muscles, good balance and sensory awareness are vital to prevent falls from happening, as so often the actual recovery from fracture can be more traumatic than the osteoporosis itself. Certain exercises have been found to be ideal for improving co-ordination and balance and they actually decrease the risk of fracture due to falling. These include alternate forward lunges and travelling side squats.

THE EFFECTS OF PHYSICAL ACTIVITY ON THE HEART

Like any other muscle in the body the heart needs to be worked in order to be strengthened. During the menopause, as we are no longer protected by the effect of oestrogen, it is not unusual for increased amounts of low-density lipoprotein (LDL), the bad cholesterol, to increase the risk of CHD. The more we exercise aerobically (increasing our oxygen intake), the stronger and more efficient our heart becomes. Improvements include the ability of the heart to beat slower and to pump larger quantities of blood through with each contraction during a resting state. At the same time, more oxygen is circulated through the body and exchanged into tissues and working muscles. Of course, we must remember that other factors such as nutrition, stress levels, smoking and general lifestyle behaviours do come into play. Obviously, the healthier the lifestyle we adopt, the more likely it is that physical activity, performed at the correct duration and intensity, will actually help to reduce LDL, increase high-density lipoprotein (HDL), the good cholesterol, normalise weight, mediate blood pressure and subsequently help to protect us from CHD.

There are many reasons why exercise and physical activity are vital throughout our whole lives. However with the myriad of physiological and psycho-social changes that take place during the menopause, the importance of physical activity cannot be over-emphasised, as you will see from the list of benefits that follow:

The benefits of exercise during the menopause

Exercise increases:

- high-density lipoproteins
- oxygen transport
- aerobic capacity
- circulation
- bone mass density
- reaction time/co-ordination
- well-being

Exercise decreases:

- low-density lipoproteins
- heart disease risk
- blood pressure
- body fat percentage
- anxiety
- depressed mood
- the effects of stress

THE PSYCHOLOGICAL EFFECTS OF PHYSICAL ACTIVITY

For each individual woman the experience of the menopause will be very different. Whilst for some this may be a positive time of liberation and freedom, for others the variety of physiological and psycho-social changes that occur may be encountered with fear and anxiety. The menopause will affect every woman differently. Personality, mood status, anxiety thresholds, culture, social experience, expectations and fear of ageing are but a few of the factors that make each woman's journey through the menopause very individual. Although research investigating exercise and the menopause has tended to focus on the physiological effects, more recently the effects of physical activity on psychological processes of this life-stage have been investigated.

Major studies have found that for active men and women of all ages depressed mood, clinical depression and anxiety may be reduced by physical exercise. However, during the menopause, things shift. This life stage is now recognised as a time of social change when external circumstances may in fact be responsible for psychological trauma. It has also been found that depressed mood during the menopause may be linked to past experiences of depression, personality and coping ability rather than to reduced oestrogen levels. Depressed mood may also be associated with other menopausal characteristics such as hot flushes, nightsweats and the resultant lack of sleep. Although it has not yet been established that exercise can reduce hot flushes, significant associations have been found between improvements in well-being and reductions of depressed mood in exercising women.

Whether you are an experienced exerciser or new to the concept of exercising for health, it is never too late to gain the benefits of an active lifestyle. Furthermore, the advantages that physical activity may bring will be more than welcomed during the menopause transition. You've taken your first step by reading this far, so now let us put these words into action – let's get physical.

GETTING STARTED

Health check

When I first consult a new client of menopausal status, I will always strongly recommend a series of health assessments to evaluate that client's health and fitness. I take these steps regardless of exercise experience and I would recommend these assessments to you if have not previously had them. Remember, if you are new to exercising or if you are in any doubt at all about your fitness, then do make a point of visiting your GP. Before you go any further, it is also vital that you are not in any pain whatsoever whilst exercising: aim for safety and effectiveness every time.

1 Get a baseline measurement of your Bone Mineral Density (BMD). You can do this through your GP or at a health clinic in a hospital. I recommend Duel-energy x-ray absorptiometry (DEXA) as this is recognised as the 'gold standard' of BMD measurement.

2 To measure your cholesterol, you can have a blood lipid profile which will evaluate both your LDL and HDL levels, again through your GP. If you fall into a high-risk category for CHD it may be wise to have an electrocardiogram (ECG) to monitor your heart rate under exercising conditions.

3 Identify your resting heart rate (table 1) and from there calculate your own training heart rate (table 2). I will explain this in detail later.

4 Check that you are taking the correct amount of calcium, fish oils, vitamin D and phytoestrogens (this you can do through the WNAS).

PHYSICAL ACTIVITY AND HORMONE REPLACEMENT THERAPY (HRT)

As an exercise and health practitioner I have worked with many menopausal women, and I have become aware that making decisions about HRT treatment and physical activity participation may be very confusing. In many instances, HRT and physical activity are both chosen. This is fine, but I do stress that you really have to understand the choices that are available and not just accept HRT as the magic answer. In many cultures the menopause is recognised as a natural transition and a time of liberation and wisdom and HRT is not even an option. We, in the Western world however, tend to be 'treated' for the menopause, with the cure being HRT. Is this really what we have come to accept?

As I have explained, exercise may increase bone density, decrease the risk of CHD and improve well-being and depressed mood; however, it has not been found to reduce hot flushes. Correct nutrition has been found to help in the reduction of the hot flush. If you are in a low-risk category for CHD and osteoporosis, you are experiencing depressed mood and do not wish to take HRT, the option of regular, moderate, physical activity is preferable.

PHYSICAL ACTIVITY VS. STRUCTURED EXERCISE PROGRAMMING

Firstly, before you begin to get active, I would like you to realise that you do not have to go to the gym three times a week, undress in a communal changing room and compete with younger women in a high-impact aerobics class with music that you can't stand. Of course there are those who prefer to participate in exercise classes or to work-out in the gym and that is great; however, although for many people the gym is a motivational tool, for others it may be one of the biggest barriers to exercising.

Remember that saying, 'no pain no gain'? Well, you can forget it! It is now understood and accepted that exercising for health and exercising for fitness are two different concepts. If your goals are to improve your health, the Health Education Authority (HEA) strongly recommend active living as an alternative to structured exercise programming. This is all about bringing physical activity into daily life and really enjoying it. It is not about 'having to' but about 'wanting to' and the great thing is there are no rules. If you want to dance alone in your living room for 10 minutes to your favourite music, now is the time to do it. The HEA now recommend 30 minutes of moderate aerobic activity a day for improved health and the ACSM now recognise that it is possible to divide this 30 minutes into separate sessions and still achieve similar health benefits to a single 30-minute bout of exercise. Later on I shall be explaining how to monitor the intensity of your work so that you know if you are achieving these health benefits.

HOW MUCH IS ENOUGH?

There could be a million and one reasons why you should not get active. 'I have no time', 'I'm too busy', or you simply feel embarrassed. You may not have enjoyed exercising in the past or feel too tired. In many cases it may be easier to make an excuse that fully justifies not starting than to find the right reason to get started. The fact is that, as with most things, we have to want the benefits of exercise, otherwise the excuses will always be the reality. One question often asked is, 'how much is enough?' to which the appropriate response may be 'how little is enough?' As I explained earlier, the recommended quantity of activity for improved health benefits is only 30 minutes a day and this can be divided into smaller time spans. Naturally, if you are aiming to really increase your fitness levels then your goals may be very different. Do whatever you enjoy – home is a great place to start.

STRENGTHENING THE HEART

Assuming that you have followed the steps outlined in the health check then you will have a good indicator of your bone mineral density, blood lipid levels, resting heart rate and calcium intake. If you are at low risk from osteoporosis and CHD then you can assume that your exercise regime will help to maintain that status. You may be able to participate in most activities, but if you are new to exercise or returning after a break, start slowly and build up. For example, your 10-minute walk would be on flat ground rather than climbing uphill. If you are at a higher risk from CHD and/or osteoporosis, then you will have to follow the dietary recommendations to the letter and become dedicated to your chosen daily exercise regime. In this instance, you will still be taking a preventive measure by being active, but some exercises may be inappropriate for your condition, as you will see. Let us assume for the moment that you are in good health and at low risk from CHD and osteoporosis. How would you begin? Well, you are now aiming to benefit from the effects of regular, moderate, aerobic activities. Working aerobically means that you are working at an intensity that will allow your body to utilise the available oxygen; it is this oxygen that provides all of these great health benefits. So your aim here is to choose activities that can be sustained from five minutes to one hour.

Begin by making three individual lists of aerobic activities

List 1 – all of the everyday activities that you really enjoy doing and that you will find easy to make a part of everyday life, from climbing the tube escalator to gardening.

List 2 – the activities that you have never tried but would like to, such as a day's hiking, salsa classes or yoga.

List 3 – the activities that you really do not enjoy and are not interested in trying at all.

The activities in List 1 will eventually become a part of your everyday life. They may be already, but you have not yet noticed. What is important here is that you really become as active as possible, whenever possible. Try to identify situations that could make you more naturally active. Get up and walk (or cycle if possible) to the shops or park the car two blocks away from home and walk the rest of the way. If you use the bus, then get off two stops earlier and walk the rest of the way. Try treating housework as a 'work-out'. Gardening and digging are now considered to be great for bone strengthening. After a while, these activities will all become a natural part of your active day.

The activities in List 2 may need a little more planning! Take, for example, the salsa class. I have a client who could never find the appropriate aerobic class, the music was always too loud and too fast, the routines were never simple enough and the teacher never interested, and so on. After putting herself through major feelings of guilt because she could not conform to the traditional concept of 'working out', she realised that it didn't have to be this way and that it was really necessary to enjoy being active. She took time to find salsa classes that were held regularly in her area. She enrolled and is still enjoying them and really appreciating the health benefits. You too can apply this to your life. If its walking you love, then check out the National Trust cross country walks. The fun part about this is that you may discover activities that you never expected to participate in.

The activities in List 3 are best forgotten. It is much better to focus on the exercises you enjoy.

Frequency and duration

Armed with Lists 1 and 2, you can start to devise your own personal programme. If you are a complete beginner, then start by spending 10 minutes on your favourite activity for four days a week. From here you can gradually build up to between 30–40 minutes a day for five to six days a week. You will be surprised at how enjoyable it is to achieve this. However, Rome was not built in a day, so remember to take it slowly.

An example may be:

Week 1 – three days at 10 minutes

Week 2 – three days at 10 minutes

Week 3 – three days at 12 minutes

Week 4 – four days at 12 minutes ... and so on until you build up to
        the required amount.

Intensity

Intensity measures how hard you are working when exercising aerobically on a regular basis for sustained periods of time. In your training zone this will usually be between 50–80 per cent of your maximum heart rate (table 2). A simple check to measure your intensity is the talk test: if you can talk or sing comfortably whilst exercising, then you are not working too hard. For a more accurate training zone calculation you can use the simple training formula at the end of chapter 14 (table 2). What you are aiming for is for your heart to be beating a little faster than when you are resting and to be slightly hotter than when at rest. Being in this exercising state may make you feel a little uncomfortable, but this is fine as long as you are not in any pain. It is important that you take it slowly to start with and that after exercising you allow time for your body to cool down back to its pre-exercising state. As you become fitter and stronger you will find it easier to do more each session.

There are many aerobic activities to chose from. However, if you happen to be in the high-risk category for CHD, I would recommend that you liaise closely with your GP and/or with a clinical personal trainer who will be able to monitor your work intensity and progress.

The power of walking

Regular walking at the right pace acts as a great form of exercise for strengthening the heart, improving BMD, losing weight and delivering available oxygen to the working muscles. It's easy, you can walk alone or start a programme with a friend and it does not cost a penny! When walking at a brisk pace, you will find that your heart rate rises and you may feel a little breathless. As you progress, you will find it easier to introduce new challenges such as longer distances and hill walking.

If you exercise aerobically for five–six times a week for 30 minutes, at the correct intensity, you must allow 12 weeks for cardiorespiratory improvements.

Building those bones

To improve bone density it is necessary to take part in weight-bearing activities at least three times a week. These activities include:
- walking at a brisk pace (legs up to the hips)

- jogging (legs up to the hips)
- dancing (legs up to the hips)

- skipping (legs up to the hips)
- walking upstairs at steady pace (legs up to hips)
- resistance training (upper and lower body and spine)
- carrying shopping or heavy bags (upper body)
- digging the garden (upper body)
- walking with a rucksack with a light weight inside (spine).

As you can see, most of these activities are also aerobic. However, you may really like swimming, which is not weight-bearing but is aerobic, so then you would have to include, say, a brisk walk to the pool for your weight-bearing activity.

All of these exercises are good for strengthening bone. However, if your bone mineral density is below average, then beware. Avoid exercises which include bending and rotating through the spine, which may be a vulnerable area, and balancing positions that may induce a fall. Additionally, osteoporotic bone may be extremely fragile and very brittle, so that carrying too much excess weight could actually cause a fracture. In this instance it is always advisable to liaise with your doctor before participating in what may be potentially harmful activities.

AVOID:

- leaving clutter around that you may trip over (books/leads and wires)
- certain yoga positions (head/shoulder stands and spinal flexion and rotation)
- high-impact movements (jogging, skipping, rebounding)
- balanced positions (cycling, skipping, certain yoga positions)
- standing exercises performed without the use of a wall for balance (squats/lunges).

If you do weight-bearing exercise three times weekly, you must allow at least one year for improvements in bone density, and other lifestyle factors may also play a major role, especially diet and nutritional state.

Table 1

Resting heart rate

To be monitored on three consecutive mornings before rising.
To take your pulse, place two fingers on your wrist, palm side up.
Time a six-second count and write down the number of beats.
Multiply this number by 10 to get a one-minute count.
Repeat on mornings two and three.

Add up the three totals and then divide by three.
This is your resting heart rate. For most healthy women the resting
heart rate is between 75 and 84 beats per minute (bpm).

Table 2

Simplified training heart rate formula

---

220 – AGE = maximum heart rate (MHR)
MHR x 50% = 50% of MHR

Example

220 – 50 = 170 (MHR)
170 x 50 % = 85

So, whilst exercising in your training zone, you will be working between
85 bpm and 136 bpm. Any higher than this and you will not be gaining
the benefit of the available oxygen.

Examples of bone-strengthening exercises
for normal bone density exercisers.

Wrist: wall pushes
  1 Stand 2 feet (half a metre) from a wall
  2 Place hands on the wall at shoulder width
  3 Push hands and wrists into the wall as if you are trying to move the
      wall
  4 Hold for three seconds then release and repeat eight times.

Spine: lower back extension
  1 Lie face down on the floor
  2 Place hands palms down on your buttocks
  3 Keeping your eyes on the floor, very gently lift your upper torso
      away from the floor with your feet stuck firmly on the floor – avoid
      moving through the neck as you are only aiming to work the mus-
      cles at the lumbar spine.
  4 You may only be able to lift up by three–four inches (8 cms) but
      this is fine. Release back to the resting position and repeat when
      ready
  5 Repeat eight times.

Ankles: heel lifts

1 Stand 1 foot (35 cms) away from the wall
2 Place feet shoulder-width apart
3 Slowly lift your heels away from the floor
4 Hold this position for one second then lower your heels
5 As your heels lower to the floor, slightly bend your knees to distract pressure from the lower back
6 Repeat eight times.

Fall prevention travelling squats

1 Stand behind and hold onto the back of a chair
2 Place both feet firmly on the floor
3 Take your right leg out to the side of your body and place your foot on the floor so that it is a few feet away from the left foot
4 As you do this, you will have to bend both knees so that you are now in a pliée squat position
5 Hold for a few seconds and then bring your right foot back to the mid-line of your body
6 Repeat this exercise on the left leg and then alternate right to left 16 times.

Never underestimate the benefits of exercise. As well as helping to improve our health prospects, it also helps us to maintain our zest for life.

13
THE BENEFITS
OF RELAXATION

Our lifestyle in the 1990s and the demands that life places on us are quite different from the experience of past generations. The average woman has so much more on her plate, without necessarily having the support network of bygone days. The net result of the excessive demands on our time and our attention may leave us feeling stressed.

While a certain amount of stress may be good for us, since it tends to keep us mentally on our toes, there comes a point when stress can be overwhelming. Feeling stressed-out for any length of time can take its toll, both physically and mentally. It has long been medically acknowledged that stress can affect the hormone cycle and in some studies of menstruating women it has been shown to suppress ovulation. When the menopause descends on us, bringing additional changes and strains, we need to learn to improve our ability to cope with life's stresses – which are unlikely to go away.

66 Debra's Story 99

Debra is a 52-year-old wife and mother from Cardiff. She heard about the WNAS programme at a time when she was on HRT but still feeling very low.

'I first came to hear of the WNAS through an article in the local press. It interested me because the person about whom it was written had suffered severe menopausal symptoms and had been greatly helped by the WNAS programme. My own symptoms were really a continuation of premenstrual symptoms, which I had endured for many years. It had not occurred to me that a nutritional approach would be beneficial. I had never sought help, believing that I would eventually get better!

Menopause Symptom Questionnaire

Do you suffer from any of the following? Please ensure each symptom is only ticked *once*.

DEBRA	* How many times per month	None	Mild	Moderate	Severe
1 Hot/cold flushes*		✓			
2 Facial/body flushing*		✓			
3 Nightsweats*		✓			
4 Palpitations*		✓			
5 Panic attacks*		✓			
6 Generalised aches and pains					
7 Depression				✓	
8 Perspiration		✓			
9 Numbness/skin tingling in arms and legs		✓			
10 Headaches					✓
11 Backaches		✓			
12 Fatigue				✓	
13 Irritability			✓		
14 Anxiety			✓		
15 Nervousness				✓	
16 Loss of confidence				✓	
17 Insomnia			✓	✓	
18 Giddiness/dizziness		✓			
19 Difficulty/frequency in passing water		✓			
20 Water retention		✓			

21	Bloated abdomen	✓	
22	Constipation	✓	
23	Itchy vagina	✓	
24	Dry vagina	✓	
25	Painful intercourse	✓	
26	Decreased sex drive		✓
27	Loss of concentration		✓
28	Confusion/Loss of vitality		✓

Have you noticed since the onset of the menopause:

1 Loss of height   Yes ☐ No ☑

2 Difficulty in bending   Yes ☐ No ☑

3 Increased curvature of back   Yes ☐ No ☑

Are any of the above symptoms cyclic? (i.e. come in cycles, for example on a monthly basis _____

Have you gained weight since you started the menopause?   Yes ☐ No ☑ If yes, how much _____

Do you have any other menopausal symptoms not mentioned above?   No

How long have you had menopausal symptoms?   *A continuation of pre-menstrual tension*

Did you suffer from pre-menstrual tension prior to the menopause?   Yes ☐ No ☑ If yes, for how long? 30 yrs.

Follow-up Menopause Questionnaire

Do you suffer from any of the following? Please ensure each symptom is only ticked once.

DEBRA	*How many times per month	None	Mild	Moderate	Severe
1 Hot/cold flushes*		✓			
2 Facial/body flushing*		✓			
3 Nightsweats*			✓		
4 Palpitations*		✓			
5 Panic attacks*		✓			
6 Generalised aches and pains					
7 Depression			✓		
8 Perspiration		✓			
9 Numbness/skin tingling in arms and legs					
10 Headaches			✓		
11 Backaches		✓			
12 Fatigue			✓		
13 Irritability		✓			
14 Anxiety		✓			
15 Nervousness			✓		
16 Loss of confidence			✓		
17 Insomnia			✓		
18 Giddiness/dizziness		✓			
19 Difficulty/frequency in passing water		✓			
20 Water retention		✓			

21 Bloated abdomen				✓	
22 Constipation				✓	
23 Itchy vagina				✓	
24 Dry vagina				✓	
25 Painful intercourse				✓	
26 Decreased sex drive				✓	
27 Loss of concentration				✓	
28 Confusion/Loss of vitality				✓	

About two years ago or more, my periods became irregular and as well as the usual headaches, depression and nervousness, I began having nightsweats. That year was also the start of a very stressful period in my life when three members of our family died and some minor incidents added to the stress. My headaches became constant and very oppressive for some months and I knew I had to get help as I felt that I was rapidly going downhill. I saw my doctor and asked if I could start on HRT, hoping that this would ease my headaches and depression. After about four months on HRT I felt no better, but no worse either, so I decided to contact the WNAS.

After a few weeks of starting the programme, I noticed a slight difference and very gradually I began to feel better. It certainly helped me through a very difficult time. Now, a year later, with regular exercise, a controlled diet and the supplements, my symptoms have eased considerably and I find I have much more energy. The quality of my sleep is better and I wake feeling refreshed most mornings, whereas I used to be so fatigued. I don't feel irritable any more and I have far fewer headaches. There have been two other benefits from the programme. I suffered a lot with swollen ankles for a couple of years but this has now stopped. I also had a problem with burning eyes, which often felt so tired and prickly, and this has also stopped.

I came off HRT six months ago for a trial period and as things are going so well I have not restarted it.

I hope that my experience will encourage other women to take the natural approach to the menopause and also to premenstrual syndrome. I certainly wish I had known about the WNAS a long time ago.'

Stress is also able to affect our digestive process, bringing abdominal and bowel symptoms that we may not have experienced before. When we are under considerable emotional and psychological stress, it's possible that we are more likely to develop food intolerances. Often the stress persists, the symptoms become chronic, or the individual may be passed off as neurotic or a hypochondriac – and things go from bad to worse. Ineffective treatment, or inadequate belief in the physical nature of our symptoms, often contributes further to our stress.

LEARNING THE ART OF RELAXATION

Stress and relaxation are at two opposite ends of the spectrum. When they are in balance you are coping, but when the scales tip and stress outweighs relaxation, symptoms often develop. As our lifestyle these days is far from relaxed, we should consciously protect ourselves from excess stress by learning relaxation techniques which, unlike stress, do not come naturally.

Relaxation has also been shown to influence hot flushes in a medical study conducted in 1984. They showed a 60 per cent reduction in the frequency of flushes in a group of women who were given relaxation training. A further study published in the *European Menopause Journal* in 1995 found that relaxation helped to overcome hot flushes.

But relaxing may not be as easy as it sounds. When you are feeling wound up and tense, learning to release tension from tensed muscles is an acquired skill. Once you have mastered the art, however, it can be practised at any time, requires only space and time and is free of charge!

Instead of focusing on the outside world and the problems that it brings, you will need to learn to tune-in to your body and become sensitive to its tensions. Even if you have never been taught any basic relaxation techniques, what is involved is quite simple.

You will need to wear some loose, comfortable clothes and find a warm space where you will be uninterrupted. Either lie down on a mat, on a soft carpet or on a bed. Make sure you are comfortable with the room temperature and lighting. If you like music, you can practise this relaxation technique while calming music is playing in the background. Once you feel comfortable, do the following, step-by-step:

1 Place a pillow under your head and relax your arms and your lower jaw.
2 Take a few slow deep breaths before you begin.
3 Then concentrate on relaxing your muscles, starting with the toes on one foot and then the other. Gradually work your way slowly up your body.
4 As you do so, first tense each group of muscles and then relax them, taking care to breathe deeply as you relax.
5 When you reach your head, and your face feels relaxed, remain in the relaxed position for about 15 minutes.
6 Gradually allow yourself to 'come to'.

Yoga

Yoga has been practised throughout the world for thousands of years. It works on the principle of bringing about a harmonious balance between your mind, body and soul. It is particularly effective at helping to relieve stress and stress-related conditions. To get started, it's best to attend a yoga class and then to practise the postures at home on a regular basis.

There are many good books on yoga, and there are now a few yoga videos which you might find helpful.

From the midlife survey carried out recently, we found that 19 per cent tried yoga and found it helpful.

Massage

Massage is a term used to describe a fairly ancient art of healing by touch, and if you think about it, we often subconsciously touch or rub a painful area in an attempt to bring relief. There are several different massage techniques to choose from, but essentially massage is designed to heal, relieve tension, improve circulation and help the body to rid itself of toxins.

Massage can also relieve pain by stimulating the production of brain chemicals called endorphins, the body's own painkillers, and by blocking out the transmission of pain messages by increasing the sensory input to the brain.

There are different ways of getting a regular massage, depending on your pocket and your situation. You can book an appointment with a registered masseuse, which can be quite expensive. You can enlist the help of your partner or a friend, or alternatively you can learn to self-massage, but this does have its limitations unless you have arms like Twizzle. If you enjoy being massaged but have a limited budget, you might enjoy learning how to massage by following a short course. Teaming up with another can be the cheapest way of getting a regular massage. Most local authorities have classes and there are several good books on the subject.

In the meantime, if you would like to experiment, take a few drops of an aromatherapy oil of your choice – lavender, orange and melissa are particularly relaxing – mix it with some almond oil and rub yourself in a clockwise direction on your abdomen, with stroking motions on your arms and legs, and gentle smoothing motions on your face and neck. Give your scalp and your temples a massage. Lastly, rub your ears between your thumb and forefinger, starting at the top and working your way down to the ear lobe, pulling gently at the same time. It feels wonderful and increases the circulation to your face and head.

Influencing the subconscious

There are many ways of stimulating the subconscious mind to heal the body and medical studies have been done to show that it works! It's thought that the subconscious can be influenced by suggestion and imagination: hence the placebo response that we sometimes hear about in clinical trials, where the dummy pill apparently produced an effect. There are many different methods of stimulating the subconscious mind and it's important to choose a system that you feel comfortable with, in order to achieve your objective. To find the self-help measure that you feel happy with, you may have to experiment.

At the Center for Climacteric Studies in Gainsville, Florida, Dr Morris Notelovitz has been testing non-hormonal methods of helping menopausal symptoms. One particular study, using biofeedback training, which had previously been shown to manipulate heart rate, skin responses, vascular diameter and muscle tension and had been used to help patients with migraine, was used to help overcome hot flushes.

Biofeedback is another relaxation technique. With this method a machine is often used and a deep state of relaxation achieved. The eight women on the study had never encountered biofeedback before, but were trained in the method before they started. The women were taught to consciously cool their hands for 45 seconds during a hot flush and to consciously warm their hands in between flushes. Their progress was measured on the biofeedback machine. The training period lasted for four weeks and the trial was continued for a further four weeks, with the women recording hourly records throughout the day. While the duration of each flush remained the same, the associated discomfort dropped significantly. This looks encouraging although larger, controlled studies need to be conducted.

Creative Visualization

This is a wonderfully simple and most enjoyable method of relaxation, requiring little or no training. It is perfect for those who haven't had the time to learn how to practise yoga or meditation. You lie flat on the floor, with a cushion beneath your head. Bend your knees and place your feet flat on the floor, so that you are in what is called 'the Alexander position'. Next, close your eyes, take some slow, steady breaths, and consciously relax your face, fingers and toes. When you feel comfortable, whilst still breathing slowly and steadily, you simply visualise any fantasy you fancy – or you can visualise yourself symptom-free and cool. The trick is to keep your mind on the trip in question. It seems to be an acquired skill, and one that you may have to work at. If you have a very busy mind, you may at first need to have a pen and paper handy, in order to download your thoughts. You need to do 15 or 20 minutes per day, and then gently come back to reality, rolling over onto your side prior to standing. Some patients feel so relaxed doing their creative visualisation that they fall asleep!

Pilates

Pilates is one of the most recent forms of relaxation/exercise techniques to reach our leisure centres and home videos. It has become very popular, particularly for people who cannot cope with high-impact exercise such as running and aerobics, as it offers a more gentle format, ideal for relaxation at the same time. Developed in the 1920s by the legendary physical trainer, Joseph H. Pilates, the discipline is a combination of Western and Eastern philosophies, teaching you about breathing with movement, body mechanics, balance, co-ordination, positioning of the body, spatial awareness and strength and flexibility.

Self-hypnosis

This method helps to bring about the feeling of calmness and mental agility. It is a system of implanting positive messages which have a therapeutic value. Half an hour each day can leave you feeling refreshed and in a more positive mood.

Autogenic Training

This is designed to tap into the body's own in-built powers of self-healing. It consists of repeating six different commands slowly in sequence until you reach a semi-hypnotic state. The end result is a much more relaxed and positive you – and initially requires only half an hour or so three times each week.

All these and many more relaxation techniques can be learned at specialist centres throughout the UK. It really is worth investing a little of your time in order to learn how to relax and rise above the stresses and strains of everyday life.

15

BANISHING MIDLIFE SYMPTOMS NATURALLY

We have already discussed *why* diets need to be changed in order to start ameliorating menopausal symptoms; and more specific details will be given on diet in Part Four. The importance of exercise and relaxation has been emphasised as well. So, with the information you already have, and the dietary options to follow, you should be able to make an effective start on banishing your menopausal symptoms in a natural and healthy way.

FLUSHES

We now know that hot flushes are triggered by a number of factors: external heat like an over-warm room, sunshine, heavy blankets and hot-water bottles, alcohol, tea, coffee and possibly spicy foods. The circulation of women experiencing flushes is much more sensitive to environmental factors, rather than being under their own control, and it is this sensation of being out of control that is one of the most detested phenomena among menopausal women. Flushes are more likely to be troublesome at the start of the menopause and in some women can persist for many years.

Set aside 15–20 minutes per day for formal relaxation. By doing so you can reduce your hot flushes by 60 per cent (see also Chapter 13, The Benefits of Relaxation).

You can help to minimise flushing by implementing some of the following advice:

1 Include a good serving of the following plant oestrogens in your diet every day: soy products, including So Good soy milk with cereals or mixed fruit as a fruit shake, tofu and silken tofu blended with fruit, golden linseeds, chick peas, lentils, mung beans, alfalfa, sunflower, pumpkin and sesame seeds and green and yellow vegetables.

2 Cut down on the number of hot drinks you consume, especially tea and coffee.
3 Don't have a hot drink on an empty stomach.
4 Avoid hot, spicy foods.
5 Use several thin layers of bedclothes rather than one heavy duvet.
6 Avoid spending time out-of-doors in the heat of a summer's day.
7 Wear several thin layers of clothing rather than thick clothes, even if it's cold.
8 Control the temperature inside your home so that you feel comfortable.
9 Keep your alcohol consumption down to a minimum.
10 Take a supplement of Novogen Red Clover – a natural dietary isoflavone food supplement for women. Phytoestrogen-rich, it delivers 40 mg of isoflavones per tablet, and allows us to top up on naturally occurring phytoestrogens.

Make the changes above, follow the dietary changes designed to help you get the best out of natural oestrogens (see page 137), and exercise regularly. Exercise helps to improve your body's control of circulation and smooth out some of the mood swings that occur in women troubled by hot flushes. Don't panic if you do not experience immediate relief: it may take three months for you to feel the full effect of this method of controlling flushes.

VAGINAL DRYNESS

This problem is related to oestrogen withdrawal and can be helped by factors other than oestrogen-replacement therapy. Studies published in some respected medical journals have shown potentially beneficial changes in the cells lining the vagina from a diet rich in soya flour, linseeds and sprouted red clover and from the use of ginseng. Other dietary sources of similar oestrogen-like compounds exist (see page 122).

A combination of dietary changes, exercise and the use of the nutritional supplements for other problems associated with the menopause help to improve vaginal secretions in some women. A study conducted by Australian researchers at MONASH university on menopausal women using soya, red clover and linseeds, showed that they were able to bring about the same changes in the lining of the vagina as in women taking HRT. Patience is required as it does take several months to influence our function.

Lubricants are very important in the short term. The traditionally recommended KY jelly is a water-based lubricant useful at times of sexual activity. More recently, a vaginal gel, Replens, given by use of an applicator, produces effective vaginal lubrication and only needs to be inserted three times each week. It is available over the counter from the chemist.

During the menopause and into the postmenopause, sexual stimulation does still increase vaginal moisture. However, instead of taking less than a minute it takes approximately five. So tell your partner that he should whisper sweet nothings into your ear for a little longer!

And try the following:

1 Follow the Option Three diet on page 246 for three months.
2 Include the oestrogen-like foods and drinks in your diet as these have been shown to help the vaginal tissues. The list of these foods and drinks starts on page 147.
3 Take a supplement of Novogen Red Clover – a natural dietary isoflavone food supplement for women. A phytoestrogen-rich supplement, it delivers 40 mg of isoflavones per tablet which allows us to top up on naturally occurring phytoestrogens.
4 Do pelvic-floor exercises regularly and make sure you get three or four good general exercise sessions every week.
5 Try some extra foreplay before actual intercourse. If you find it hard to get started, a massage might help. There are some lovely aromatherapy oils available. You only need a few drops of the aromatherapy oil mixed with some almond oil which you can buy at the chemist. Ask your partner to give you a gentle massage – and you might like to return the favour!
6 Don't be afraid to use lubricants like Replens or KY jelly when you feel you need to. If you have enjoyed a fulfilling sex life, do all within your power to preserve it.

URINARY SYMPTOMS

The symptoms of urinary frequency, urgency and incontinence become increasingly common in postmenopausal women, which can be both distressing and embarrassing. One group of American experts recently concluded that though HRT seems to help stress-incontinence, the amount of actual fluid lost is no less as a result of treatment. More effective treatments include surgery for those who are severely affected and have a prolapse. Exercises to strengthen the muscles of the pelvic floor can be very effective as is sometimes the use of a ring pessary inserted into the vagina, although this is only suitable for older women.

The symptoms of urinary frequency are often made worse by a high intake of the caffeine from tea and coffee. Urgency and mild discomfort can occasionally be due to dietary factors. The term 'irritable bladder syndrome' is used to describe this problem, providing infection has been ruled out as a cause. We have seen a few such women whose symptoms of urgency and discomfort have improved with the avoidance of a variety of foods in the same way that the symptoms of irritable bowel syndrome can also improve.

So you can try the following:

1 Practise pelvic-floor exercises three or four times each day as described in the general recommendations.
2 Avoid tea and coffee and use the alternatives suggested on page 104.
3 Try following the Option Three diet on page 246 for three months to see whether it makes any difference.
4 Concentrate particularly on a diet high in phytoestrogens, those oestrogen-like foods that are listed on page 147.
5 If there is little improvement after three months, then consult your doctor to examine the possibilities of having a surgical repair.

Interestingly, the tissues of the bladder, urethra and vagina are extremely sensitive to oestrogens. As plant phytoestrogens are excreted in the urine, they will come into contact with these areas and may therefore be particularly likely to help with these symptoms. Just changing from a high-fat, low-fibre diet to a more healthy one and not using antibiotics helps increase the amount of excreted oestrogens in the urine and reduce the amount lost in the faeces.

HEADACHES

These are variably reported as being associated with the menopause. Many women find that their migraines lessen or disappear at this time but for some they may get worse and for others tension headaches may begin.

Migraine headaches which are intermittent, often severe, always associated with nausea or vomiting, and usually associated with visual disturbance or light sensitivity, can respond well to dietary changes. Certain foods rich in the chemical 'amine' are frequent migraine-triggers. Try cutting these foods out of your diet. They include cheese, wine and most other alcoholic beverages, chocolate, yeast extract, pickled foods and oranges.

Tension headaches are less influenced by diet, alhough tea and coffee sometimes play a part and some women with persistent headaches seem to benefit from cutting out bread and other sources of grain from the diet. Anyone with persistent headaches should always check with their doctor and have their blood pressure checked.

Try the following:

1 Cut out the amine-based foods listed above that can trigger headaches.

2 Avoid tea and coffee, bearing in mind that your headaches may get worse while you go through the withdrawal phase, which may last anything from a few days to a few weeks.

3 Try eating some ginger, either root or crystallised, if you feel the headache coming on. During a headache the blood vessels constrict. Ginger, a very old remedy, has the opposite effect: it makes the blood vessels dilate and therefore can often cancel out the headache altogether. Although I have never seen any clinical trials using ginger for headaches, we have had a lot of success with it over the years, so it must be worth a try.

4 Practise either yoga or relaxation techniques if you feel your headaches are stress related. Learning how to cope with stress can make the world of difference to how you feel. Read the chapter on relaxation and work out a programme for yourself to practise on a regular basis.

DEPRESSION

Although depression is an associated symptom of the menopause, it's one that is likely to be influenced by more than just a change in hormones. Medical opinion is divided as to how often depression is due to hormonal change and how much to other physical and psychological factors.

A youngish woman with an early menopause, severe oestrogen withdrawal and plagued by hot flushes has every reason to feel depressed and will probably feel much better physically and psychologically with HRT. On the other hand, some researchers have related the presence of depression to stresses in the woman's life and in particular the stress of trying to fulfil too many functions. Juggling the identities of mother, lover, wage-earner and carer of ageing parents takes its toll and for many the result is depression. Lack of exercise can also be depressing. Indeed, a trial on a group of women of one hour's aerobic exercise three times a week for nine weeks had a marked beneficial effect on mood comparable to an antidepressant. (It also helps physical fitness and is likely to reduce the risk of heart-disease and improve bone strength.)

Lack of some nutrients can also be a factor in depression. Studies in depressed adults of both sexes and various ages have revealed that a mild to moderate lack of one or more of the B-group vitamins was found in 50 per cent of them. Women with PMS will probably have a low level of the mineral magnesium. Supplements of both the vitamins B and magnesium can help to improve mood in certain groups although, as far as we know, postmenopausal women have not been specifically studied. But it would seem worth a try especially if one or more of these risk factors applies to you:

- A high intake of alcohol: more than 14 units each week
- Dependence upon convenience foods with a poor intake of fresh vegetables, meat, fish or good quality vegetarian proteins
- A history of PMS
- Symptoms such as cracking at the corners of your mouth, a sore tongue, recurrent mouth ulcers or redness and greasiness at the sides of your nose – all possible features of vitamin B deficiency.

We have found vitamins B and magnesium sometimes helpful but again they are best considered alongside dietary and exercise measures.

Try the following:

1 Take three or four sessions of aerobic exercise per week. If you haven't the time to get out to exercise, then try one of the Y Plan videos at home. There are more details about these in the chapter on exercise.

2 Make time for yourself each day, either to go for a walk or to practise 20 minutes' relaxation, such as creative visualisation. See page 186 for details.

3 Follow the Option Three diet on page 246 for three months to see whether your depression is food-related. It may well be that a complete change in diet will help enormously.

4 Take some nutritional supplements that include B vitamins and magnesium for an initial three-month period. An example of this is Gynovite which you can read about on pages 119 and 153.

5 St John's Wort has been used to treat depression for more than two thousand years, and it now accounts for half of all the prescriptions for depression in Germany. In the UK, demand has increased following a report in the *British Medical Journal* on its efficacy. The menopause brings with it many physical and psychological changes which very often place unnecessary strain on the lives of menopausal women. A German study on 111 menopausal women with libido problems showed that a 12-week

course of St John's Wort restored libido levels in 60 per cent of the women and alleviated 80 per cent of psychological symptoms associated with the menopause, including depression, irritability, inner tension and anxiety. The recommended dosage is up to 300 mcg three times a day.

ANXIETY AND
INSOMNIA

These symptoms can be related to frequent and severe hot flushes. When this is the case, they can respond to HRT and usually respond well to our programme, as they can be aggravated by certain dietary factors and nutritional imbalances. If hot flushes prevent you from getting a good night's sleep then it's not surprising that your stress-tolerance will be low the next day.

Try the following:

1 First follow the recommendations to help hot flushes.
2 If you are still menstruating and your anxiety levels are worse in the run-up to your period, supplements of the B vitamins and magnesium may help. If you have finished menstruation, you might find that taking one of the suggested supplements will speed up the recovery process. It is worth a try. The supplements suggested are listed on page 120.
3 Relaxation techniques, yoga and breathing exercises are all potentially helpful. When you are feeling anxious, breathing too rapidly alters the body chemistry by removing too much carbon-dioxide. This has the effect of aggravating anxiety tendencies. Breathing exercises can help.
4 Follow the Option Three diet on page 246 for three months, making sure that you cut out all the stimulants such as tea, coffee, chocolate, cola and alcohol. Use the suggested alternatives.
5 Take plenty of exercise, three to four sessions each week to the point of breathlessness. If you can get out to exercise, all well and good. If not, put on an exercise video at home and go for it! See the chapter on exercise.
6 Take the herb Valerian, sold as Valerina Night and Day. Valerina Day is a traditional herbal remedy for the symptomatic relief of tenseness, irritability and the stresses of modern living. Valerina Night helps to promote sleep naturally.

7 Kava Kava is becoming an increasingly popular herb for relieving anxiety and promoting natural sleep without the side effects of sleeping tablets.

FATIGUE

This is an even more contentious symptom. While it might improve with HRT, don't count on it unless your symptoms are only associated with nightsweats and the resulting insomnia.

In women who are still menstruating, lack of iron is a common cause of fatigue. In the late-forties age group, anaemia is less of a problem but may still affect two to three per cent of women. You can still lack iron without being anaemic: this is best detected by measurement of blood level of serum ferritin (protein in the blood, which accurately reflects the level of iron in the body, not just in the haemoglobin or blood pigment). So see your doctor if you are still having periods, especially if they are still heavy. This can be a problem for some 10 per cent of perimenopausal women. Again, lack of the B vitamins or magnesium can be a factor so eat healthily and, if you fall into one of the risk groups, consider taking a supplement.

If you have any other illness or symptoms, see your doctor. Fatigue has so many possible causes that if it is severe a medical check-up is often the best way of finding out if there is anything else wrong. Diet, not just a lack of nutrients, can be a factor. There is some good evidence that undetected food allergies can be associated with fatigue (and headaches and bowel problems). Wheat and the related grains seem to be common culprits. Sometimes fatigue is a symptom of depression or stress so these may need tackling if you think it appropriate.

Try the following:

1 If you have nightsweats and insomnia, follow the recommendations on page 120.
2 If you are still menstruating, ask your doctor to measure your serum ferritin levels, which is a good test for detecting low iron stores.
3 To eliminate the possibility of food allergy being associated with your fatigue, follow the Option Three diet on page 246 for three months to see whether there is any noticeable difference.
4 Take as much regular exercise as you can. If you are really feeling shattered, this may be difficult to start with, but even five minutes every day is better than nothing. You can build up the time as your energy levels improve.

5 Take some of the vitamins and minerals suggested on page 118 to give you a boost.
6 Read a book called *Tired All The Time* by Dr Alan Stewart, and see whether you can pinpoint the underlying cause of your fatigue.
7 If you feel no better after three months, arrange an appointment with your doctor for a thorough check-up.

ACHES AND PAINS

Non-specific aches and pains are a common complaint and it's debatable whether they are actual menopause symptoms or to do with a lack of physical well-being. The enthusiasts for HRT would like to claim that it helps aches and pains. The manufacturers, however, are hesitant to do so. Certainly some women experience a substantial improvement in well-being when taking HRT and the improvement of peripheral symptoms seems to be related to the improvement in hot flushes. Interestingly, though, the oestrogen in HRT does cause a slight change in blood chemistry similar to that in pregnancy, with the production of a small amount of pregnancy zone protein (PZP). This has been extracted from the blood of pregnant women, given to non-pregnant women with rheumatoid arthritis and been found to benefit them! Some women do report feeling particularly well during pregnancy.

What is the natural alternative here? Lack of physical fitness has got to be an important factor for some women, so out of your chair and on with your walking shoes. Being overweight won't help either, so you will need to shed some pounds.

A lack of magnesium – yet again – is renowned for causing muscle cramps, so follow the dietary recommendations as they are rich in magnesium, potassium and the B vitamins, all important for muscle function. Finally, aches and pains often respond to dietary changes with the avoidance of certain foods.

Try the following:

1 Follow the Option Three diet on page 246 for at least three months.
2 If you are overweight you will need to lose weight, which you may well do anyway while on Option Three. If you are not losing weight naturally, you may have to cut your portion sizes or eat from a smaller plate!
3 Take some extra magnesium supplements as well as the suggested multi-vitamins and minerals. But be careful with extra magnesium

because, as well as being an important nutrient, it also has a laxative effect. Unless you are prone to diarrhoea, you should be able to take two or three 150 mg tablets each day; if you are constipated, you can increase the dose to four or five tablets and sort out both problems at once.

4 Regular exercise is always important, so take it easy, but make sure you do as much as you can three or four times each week.

5 Massage can soothe away aches and pains. Either treat yourself to a professional massage or persuade your partner to give you a massage several times a week. Use the lovely aromatherapy massage oils mentioned on page 185.

6 If the aches and pains persist, visit your local cranial osteopath for an evaluation. Underlying mechanical problems can really stop you making progress. Cranial osteopaths offer gentle but effective treatment, and we have had excellent feedback from patients who consulted one.

7 Glucosamine is a natural substance found abundantly in the body. It is composed of glucose and an amino acid called glutamine. Glucosamine is found in high concentrations in sea cucumber and green lipped mussel, *particularly* as glucosamine sulphate. The most efficiently absorbed form of glucosamine is glucosamine sulphate, as the presence of sulphur, a trace mineral, plays an important role in the maintenance of healthy cartilage. Several clinical studies have shown that glucosamine sulphate taken at a dose of at least 400 mg three times a day, produces significant improvements in the symptoms of pain, joint tenderness and swelling. Best effects can be achieved when taking glucosamine in conjunction with chondroitin.

WEIGHT-GAIN

Many women attribute weight-gain to the 'change'. Well, it's not really a good excuse. The metabolic rate does drop fractionally at this time but comparison of different age groups shows that on average there is something like a 1 kilo or 2 lb weight gain. A listed side-effect of HRT is weight-gain, but some researchers consider this is not really the case. However, fluid retention does seem to be common and in our survey women who had taken HRT reported an average weight-gain of 16 lbs.

In theory, being overweight or, to be more scientific about it, having lots of peripheral fat tissue, will help your body maintain its level of residual oestrogen in the postmenopausal phase. But being too plump is strongly associated with a greater risk of cancer of the womb and a slightly increased risk of breast cancer. There are also all the effects of excess weight on blood pressure, cholesterol, general fitness, mobility and self-esteem. So it doesn't pay to be overweight. Neither does it pay to be too thin. This increases the risk of osteoporosis and may not be the best for a healthy postmenopausal hormone balance.

Our advice is not to start a strict weight-loss diet just now. You will have enough to do while you are following the option of your choice, in an attempt to control your symptoms. It's important to get those symptoms under control first, before dieting. One of the added bonuses of our programme is that most people lose weight without trying. You might even find, three months down the line, you are somewhat lighter and the need to diet as such has lessened.

We have, of course, included the most important elements of a weight-loss diet into most of the options. These are:

1 Reduce the intake of fatty foods, especially those rich in saturated animal fats.
2 Cut right down on sugar, sweets, chocolate and other foods high in empty calories.
3 Limit your intake of alcohol. It's nutritionally poor and it's an easy way to increase your calories and worsen your hot flushes.
4 Eat plenty of filling, nutritious, low-calorie foods such as fresh fruit, vegetables, lean meats, fish and chicken without their skins, whole-grain bread, lower-fat dairy products and vegetarian protein.

Many women find the support of a slimming group or club is helpful, so find out what is available in your area. Your doctor may have some advice on this. There are many good slimming books, not the least of which is our own *The Zest for Life Plan*.

❝ Hilary's Story ❞

Hilary is 51 and works part time as an administrator at a university. She is married and lives with her husband in Bedfordshire. She had suffered with menopausal symptoms for about five years and, as these had recently become overwhelming, she decided it was time to do something.

'*My main symptoms were breast tenderness and I felt tired all the time. My doctor thought I should try HRT as this would also help to protect against* osteoporosis and heart disease. For a while this seemed to help but then the breast tenderness returned and I was so bloated that all my clothes were too tight, so I decided to stop taking it. About a month later I began to experience the most horrendous hot flushes, about 12 a day and another two or three at night. I had also suffered for years with headaches and migraine and for about the last two years with an unbearable skin irritation. I tried self-helping by taking some natural preparations from the health-food shop, but realised I needed more tailored advice.

This was January 1999 and my New Year's resolution was to regain control of my life. My first step towards this was to make an appointment to see Maryon Stewart at the London clinic. Prior to my first appointment I was asked to complete a Menopause Questionnaire and a seven-day diet diary, which Maryon evaluated and upon which she based her recommendations. I was asked to cut out wheat and bran because of my severe hot flushes, increase my vegetable and fruit intake and ensure a good intake of naturally ocurring oestrogens (phytoestrogens). Maryon explained the benefits of phytoestrogens and how they have a balancing effect on my own natural oestrogen. She also recommended nutritional supplements, which are formulated to alleviate symptoms of the menopause.

I found the new dietary programme really enjoyable. I would start the day with a phytoestrogen-rich muesli with soy milk and fruit; lunch was oily fish and salad and dinner consisted of fish or lean meat and fresh vegetables. I could have lots of "snacks" of nuts, seeds, fruit, raw vegetables, wheat-free snack bars and soy-milk drinks.

The results were amazing. After just two months my symptoms were largely under control and I was feeling much more positive about myself than I had for years. In addition, I had lost a few pounds in weight and had lots more energy.

At the end of the programme I had lost a stone in weight without even trying! In fact, I seemed to be eating more! My skin irritation had disappeared, I had no hot flushes and headaches were a thing of the past. I felt like a new person.'

BOWEL PROBLEMS

Constipation, bloating, abdominal discomfort and sometimes diarrhoea are common problems in women of all ages. Strictly speaking these are not part of menopausal symptoms proper but deserve a mention here as they are so common. These are the main symptoms of irritable bowel syndrome, where the bowel is over-sensitive, resulting in episodes of spasm of the muscles of the bowel wall. Diet and stress are now recognised as the two most important factors in this common condition.

There is now an acknowledged association between bowel problems and a variety of gynaecological problems, including infertility. What happens in the bowel will certainly have some influence on hormone metabolism. Our experience is that women with both PMS and menopausal symptoms seem to fare a lot better if co-existing bowel problems are also tackled simultaneously with their other symptoms.

Anyone with severe pain, blood in the stool, weight-loss or who has only recently developed symptoms should check with their doctor. The advice that follows is suitable for those with constipation or irritable bowel syndrome but not if there is some other problem.

Try the following:

1 Cut down on tea, especially if you are constipated: it can slow down bowel transit rate. Coffee can speed it up.

2 Eat plenty of fibre-rich foods, especially fresh fruit and vegetables.

3 Don't eat bran. That's right, don't eat bran. Although it's helpful for some, its effects are too unpredictable. If you can take it, eat oats and oat bran.

4 Take a fibre supplement. Your doctor may prescribe something but our favourite is golden linseeds which are available in most health-food shops. As well as being a good source of fibre, they also have some natural oestrogen-like properties. A reasonable daily amount is one or two tablespoons with some breakfast cereal or fruit and yoghurt.

5 If a further laxative is needed, a supplement of magnesium is safe, effective, old-fashioned and has some interesting properties of possible benefit to menopausal symptoms. A reasonable dose is 300 mg increasing up to 600 mg if necessary. This can be taken in the form of magnesium tablets, liquid milk of magnesia or multi-vitamins containing magnesium.

More information and advice on tackling irritable bowel syndrome can be found in our book called *No More IBS!* If bowel symptoms do not respond to the above measures within four weeks then you should undoubtedly see your doctor.

66 Lorraine's Story 99

Lorraine, aged 50 from Gloucestershire, contacted the WNAS in 1997 when she realised that she was suffering as a result of HRT.

'By the age of 50, I was experiencing nightsweats, had developed a dry vagi-

na, and my memory had become atrocious. I had also been diagnosed as having irritable bowel syndrome (IBS), with daily symptoms including severe wind, bloating and constipation.

My doctor prescribed various different HRT preparations, none of which suited me. The worst side-effects were painful tender breasts, breakthrough bleeding, headaches and weight gain. It occurred to me that I had to find a natural alternative so my first port of call was the book shop, where I came across the first edition of this book called Beat the Menopause without HRT by Maryon Stewart and the title said it all! I avidly read the book – it was like reading an account of my own symptoms – which inspired me to contact the WNAS to speak to a nutritionist.

I wrote a brief letter to the WNAS and they sent me a Menopause Questionnaire and seven-day diet diary. The questionniare enabled me to give the nutritionist a detailed account of my symptoms. I carefully completed all the forms and returned them to the WNAS, who promptly phoned to arrange an appointment for me to speak to Maryon Stewart.

Maryon explained why she wanted me to cut out all wheat and bran and, although a little hesitant, I cleared the cupboards and stocked up with oat cakes and rye bread! There was a noticeable improvement when I cut out the wheat – I experienced fewer night sweats and hot flushes. After four months, my menopausal symptoms were virtually non-existent, and my IBS had gone. Maryon suggested that I introduce French bread (made with French flour) which did not present a problem, and meant I had more flexibility with my diet.

I increased my phytoestrogen intake by drinking soy milk every day, which really grew on me! I invested in Maryon's latest book The Phyto Factor which explains in lay terms how phytoestrogens not only reduce menopausal symptoms, but also reduce the risk of some cancers while increasing bone density. The book contains phyto-rich recipes which inspired me to experiment with soy and tofu!

The benefits to my health from enrolling on the WNAS programme have been immense, and if I hadn't taken my own health in my hands, I would still be undergoing HRT and suffering from IBS. My husband says he's never seen me look so well. We are both delighted that my libido returned whilst on the WNAS programme, which has not only helped our relationship, but also my self-esteem. A big thanks to the WNAS.'

SKIN PROBLEMS

Skin-thinning does really occur with the menopause and is partly due to the decline in oestrogen. Skin quality is also very much influenced by diet, circulation and local applications of good moisturisers.

Lack of certain nutrients can influence it in the following ways:

- A lack of B vitamins can result in red, greasy patches at the sides of your nose, peeling of your lips or cracking at the corners of your mouth.
- A lack of zinc can also cause red greasy skin with dry scaly patches on your face and body.
- Generally dry skin and eczema can be influenced by a lack of essential fatty acids, or EFAs found in evening primrose oil. Some women benefit from its use and this should always be combined with a very healthy diet.
- Lack of vitamin C can also lead to skin-thinning, easy bruising and delayed healing. The lack should not occur unless you are eating very little fresh fruit and vegetables. It is more likely to be a problem in smokers and older men.

Anything that stimulates blood-flow to the skin is likely to improve its quality. This could be exercise, a massage, some sun-bathing or just getting out-of-doors on a winter's day to put a bit of colour in your cheeks.

Try the following:

1 Follow the option of your choice (see pages 217–259) for three months.
2 Take some vitamins and minerals and, if your skin is dry or you suffer with eczema, use Efamol evening primrose oil or Epogam.
3 Take regular exercise.
4 Use a good moisturiser on your face and a lotion enriched with vitamin E on your body. Blackmores Laboratories make an excellent range of reasonably priced creams and lotions which contain only natural ingredients, herbs and vitamins.
5 If the skin on your body is persistently dry, try using some mineral oil in the bath. Alpha Keri is available at the chemist and also on prescription from your doctor.
6 Read *The Natural Health Bible*, a WNAS publication which covers 120 common male and female conditions, including skin complaints. It provides information about the condition, what your doctor has to offer and what you can do naturally through diet and nutritional supplements.

THRUSH

Vaginal infection with the yeast *Candida albicans* is a common problem and most women will have experienced at least one episode of it by the time they reach the menopause. Usually it becomes less of a problem by the time of the menopause but because it's so common and has recently been so widely popularised, it deserves a mention.

There are several types of *Candida* but *albicans* is by far the most common. It is also responsible for nappy rash, thrush in the mouth, under the breasts and in other moist dark parts of our bodies. Thrush is not a serious infection but it's very annoying, producing vaginal irritation and a sticky white discharge. About 20 per cent of the normal population carry a small amount of *Candida* around with them, usually in their mouths, in their bowels or on the surface of their skin. It's quite happily sitting there doing no harm and only becomes a problem when the body's defences are reduced. This can happen after a course of antibiotics which can kill off the healthy bacteria normally present in the vagina that help to protect it from *Candida* and other infections.

Diabetes, steroid drugs and the oral contraceptive pill can all increase the risk of *Candida*. This was a considerable problem with the early oral contraceptive pill which was high in oestrogen. Today it is hardly a problem with the low- and very-low-dose pills that are available. In theory HRT could increase the risk of thrush but usually this is not the case.

A lot has recently been written about the fact that thrush can also cause a whole range of symptoms including fatigue, headaches, bowel problems, skin problems and more. The scientific evidence for this is very limited. There is reasonable evidence that it can contribute to bowel problems, especially diarrhoea, following treatment with antibiotics, nettle rash and possibly eczema and psoriasis. Some women and men are also predisposed to recurrent problems with thrush because of mild deficiencies in iron, B vitamins and other nutrients. These can reduce the body's defence mechanisms enough to allow infection with *Candida*.

If thrush is a problem you can:

1 See your doctor who can prescribe local treatment with cream or pessary. If this is not enough, treatment with tablets, sometimes for several weeks, can clear thrush and remove any reservoir that may remain in the bowel.

2 Eat a diet low in sugar, sweets and alcohol as these foods can exacerbate thrush. A few women are also sensitive to yeast-rich foods. Cutting down on bread, foods with yeast extract, vinegar, pickles and alcoholic beverages can be very important, especially for those with persistent vaginal irritation or skin problems.

3 Take a multi-vitamin supplement with iron.

4 There are natural antifungal agents in most fresh vegetables, fruits, herbs and spices. Ensure you have plenty of these in your diet.

Avoiding all fruit and other forms of carbohydrate, as has been recommended by some writers, seems to us to be unnecessarily drastic.

5 Take a supplement of Acidophillus which provides a standardised quantity of the 'good' bacteria necessary for intestinal and vaginal health. Good bacteria are often disturbed if the digestive system is malfunctioning, or you have taken antibiotics. Read *The Natural Health Bible*. It provides information about the condition, what your doctor has to offer and what you can do naturally through diet and nutritional supplements.

One of the reasons why the WNAS programme is successful is that it educates you and subsequently empowers you, with your new-found knowledge, to help yourself to better health. As you are now aware, many of the symptoms that occur at the time of the menopause are not strictly related to oestrogen withdrawal. They are symptoms that would probably have occurred anyway and would have needed to be addressed sooner or later. The programme we have devised not only helps women to overcome their menopause symptoms in the short term; it also addresses other common problems such as migraine headaches, bowel problems, mood changes, anxiety syndrome and skin problems, as well as helping to prevent osteoporosis in the longer term.

For women who have been suffering with symptoms for many years, our programme is like the key to the cage in which they have been imprisoned. For the first time they are able to walk free with their health intact and, with relief, contemplate new horizons.

Part Four gives you all the information you need to work out an initial dietary programme for yourself. This, in tandem with the exercise, supplements and relaxation already discussed, is relatively new ground which has been trodden by others, who are grateful for the help they have received and have never looked back. The system we have worked out is not exclusive. It is there for the taking, so don't waste any more time in making a start.

PART FOUR

SELF-HELP

16
CHOOSING YOUR PLAN

As in many other situations in life, there are compromises to be made. There is no magic pill that will make menopausal symptoms vanish overnight and prevent osteoporosis for ever more. You will undoubtedly need to make some changes to your diet and your lifestyle to overcome your symptoms and to have the best possible chance of avoiding osteoporosis. We have already outlined some ways in which you might do this. Now we shall concentrate on individual nutritional plans.

If your symptoms are mild to moderate, there will be less effort involved than if you have severe symptoms. So that you can select the right programme to suit your individual needs, the recommendations have been divided into three options:

Option 1: General recommendations for mild sufferers
Option 2: A specialised plan for moderate sufferers
Option 3: A tailor-made programme for more severe sufferers

You will notice that on the chart that follows you are asked to assess whether your symptoms are mild, moderate or severe. Each category has a numerical score as follows:

0 = None
1 = Mild
2 = Moderate
3 = Severe

Mild   means that symptoms are present but they do not interfere with your activities. You feel all right, but are aware that some physical and emotional changes are taking place which make you feel below par.

Moderate means that symptoms are present and they do interfere with some activities, but they are not disabling. You feel below par and may even cancel arrangements. Family and close friends are aware that you are not your usual self.

Menopause Symptom Questionnaire

Do you suffer from any of the following? Please ensure each symptom is only ticked once.

MOIRA	*How many times per month	None	Mild	Moderate	Severe
1 Hot/cold flushes*	? often		✓		
2 Facial/body flushing*	?.		✓		
3 Nightsweats*	?.		✓		
4 Palpitations*	?.		✓		
5 Panic attacks*	? not very often now		✓		
6 Generalised aches and pains			✓		
7 Depression				✓+	
8 Perspiration			✓−		
9 Numbness/skin tingling in arms and legs	in hands not bad now		✓		
10 Headaches			✓		
11 Backaches			✓		
12 Fatigue				✓+	
13 Irritability			✓		
14 Anxiety				✓	
15 Nervousness				✓	
16 Loss of confidence				✓+	
17 Insomnia		✓			
18 Giddiness/dizziness floating feeling		✓			
19 Difficulty/frequency in passing water		✓			
20 Water retention		Have had some in past			

21 Bloated abdomen	✓	
22 Constipation	✓	
23 Itchy vagina	✓	
24 Dry vagina		✓+
25 Painful intercourse haven't had any for 3½ years		
26 Decreased sex drive	✓	
27 Loss of concentration	✓	
28 Confusion/Loss of vitality		✓+

Have you noticed since the onset of the menopause:

1 Loss of height   Yes ☑ No ☐
2 Difficulty in bending   Yes ☐ No ☑ but not severe
3 Increased curvature of back   Yes ☑ No ☐

Are any of the above symptoms cyclic? (i.e. come in cycles, for example on a monthly basis   Not as far as I've noticed

Have you gained weight since you started the menopause?   Yes ☑ No ☐   If yes, how much   about 12 lbs ~ 1 stone

Do you have any other menopausal symptoms not mentioned above?   ~

How long have you had menopausal symptoms?   going on for 15 years

Did you suffer from pre-menstrual tension prior to the menopause?   Yes ☑ No ☐   If yes, for how long?

Menopause Symptom Questionnaire

Do you suffer from any of the following? Please ensure each symptom is only ticked *once*.

	* How many times per month	None	Mild	Moderate	Severe
1 Hot/cold flushes*					
2 Facial/body flushing*					
3 Nightsweats*					
4 Palpitations*					
5 Panic attacks*					
6 Generalised aches and pains					
7 Depression					
8 Perspiration					
9 Numbness/skin tingling in arms and legs					
10 Headaches					
11 Backaches					
12 Fatigue					
13 Irritability					
14 Anxiety					
15 Nervousness					
16 Loss of confidence					
17 Insomnia					
18 Giddiness/dizziness					
19 Difficulty/frequency in passing water					
20 Water retention					

21 Bloated abdomen				
22 Constipation				
23 Itchy vagina				
24 Dry vagina				
25 Painful intercourse				
26 Decreased sex drive				
27 Loss of concentration				
28 Confusion/Loss of vitality				

Severe means that symptoms are not only present, they interfere with all activities. They are severely disabling and life is hard to cope with while you are experiencing them.

I have used Moira's first menopause symptom questionnaire on page 208 to demonstrate how the chart looks when it's completed. You simply decide on the severity of each symptom and tick the appropriate box. Ideally, you should complete a new chart each month so that you can compare them. (There's a blank version of this chart on page 210 for you to fill in.)

You also need to keep a daily symptomatology diary, like the one on page 213. This covers one month, and each evening before you go to bed, you should fill in one column with a number ranging from 0–3 depending on the severity of each symptom that day. This on-going record becomes very important, particularly if you are reintroducing foods to your diet in Option Three.

Read through the three options before deciding which one to follow. Make a note of your decisions on your personal nutritional programme on page 215.

HOW TO BEGIN

Once you have chosen the programme to follow you will need to sort out your record-keeping. It's important to keep accurate records as you go along as they will prove to be an immensely useful reference.

Complete the blank Menopause Symptom Questionnaire on page 210 before you begin so that you have a clear picture of your symptoms.

- Follow the specialised regime for a period of three months
- Keep a daily symptomatology diary of all your symptoms. A chart is provided on page 213 and at the end of the book
- Keep daily diaries of what you eat and drink, of exercise taken, and relaxation. Charts for these are supplied at the end of the book (pages 340–343).
- Complete another Menopause Symptom Questionnaire after three months. This can then be compared with your first chart to measure your progress. You can see how the ladies who have told their stories fared before and after on pages 18–21 and 208–209.

Menopause Symptomatology Daily Diary

Grading of symptoms

0 None
1 Mild – present but does not interfere with activities
2 Moderate – present and interferes with activities but not disabling
3 Severe – disabling. Unable to function

Date														
Hot/cold flushes*														
Facial/body flushing*														
Nightsweats*														
Palpitations*														
Panic attacks*														
Generalised aches and pains														
Depression														
Perspiration														
Numbness/skin tingling in arms and legs														
Headaches														
Backaches														
Fatigue														
Irritability														
Anxiety														
Nervousness														
Loss of confidence														

	Insomnia	Giddiness/dizziness	Difficulty/frequency in passing water	Constipation	Itchy vagina	Dry vagina	Painful intercourse	Decreased sex drive	Loss of concentration	Weight in pounds	Notes

Personal Nutritional Programme

Summary of Recommendations

Diet

1

2

3

4

5

6

7

8

9

10

11

12

Supplements

1

2

3

4

Exercise and relaxation

1

2

3

4

Points to Remember

_____

_____

_____

_____

_____

_____

_____

_____

_____

_____

_____

_____

When you have finished preparing this chart, pin it up somewhere highly visible such as on the outside of your fridge or on your kitchen noticeboard, and refer to it daily.

17

OPTION ONE: GENERAL RECOMMENDATIONS FOR MILD SUFFERERS

If you suffer from mild symptoms, or need a preventive programme to follow before your menopause, you should follow these general dietary guidelines rather than make any radical changes.

GENERAL DIETARY GUIDELINES

- Concentrate on eating foods that contain phytoestrols or phyto-oestrogens, with oestrogen-like properties. You will find a list of these on page 147.
- Reduce your intake of sugar and junk foods. This includes sugar added to tea and coffee, and in sweets, cakes, biscuits, chocolate, jam, puddings, marmalades, soft drinks containing phosphates, ice-cream and honey. Consumption of these may cause water retention and impede the uptake of essential minerals.
- Reduce your intake of salt, both added to cooking and at the table. Avoid salted foods such as salted nuts, kippers and bacon. Salt causes fluid retention and induces calcium loss from the body in the urine. LoSalt is low sodium, potassium rich and makes a good substitute without having the inherent problems associated with table salt. LoSalt is widely available from supermarkets and health-food shops. Avoid over-spicy foods as these can aggravate hot flushes.
- Eat vegetables and salads daily. Three portions of vegetables and a salad should be eaten every day, as they contain plenty of essential nutrients. Where possible use good quality vegetables, preferably organic, or try growing your own. Eat a combination of green leafy vegetables, peas, beans and lentils. These are all good sources of fibre, calcium, magnesium and other minerals.

- Eat plenty of fresh fruit, at least two servings each day. Fruit is a good source of important nutrients and a healthy way to satisfy a sweet tooth.
- Millet, buckwheat, rye and barley are high in magnesium and fibre. Oatmeal is a good source of complex carbohydrates and fibre. Eat at least one serving of cereal each day, as long as you do not get abdominal bloating as a result.
- Limit your consumption of red meat to one or two portions each week. Substitute meat with fish, poultry, peas, beans and nuts. Rice and beans also combine to form a complete protein. Meat-eaters have a lesser bone density than women who are vegetarian: animal proteins can take calcium and other minerals from bones which can then increase your chances of osteoporosis.
- Dairy products, such as milk and cheese, are excellent sources of calcium. Use low-fat versions if you need to lose or watch your weight. Drink up to one pint of milk every day. If you drink less than this, you will need to eat plenty of other calcium-rich foods. Good non-dairy sources of calcium include tinned bony fish such as sardines and salmon. Mash up the fish so that you can eat the little bones, which are extremely rich in calcium. All green vegetables, peas, beans, lentils, nuts, especially brazils, almonds and cashews and most seeds such as sesame, sunflower and pumpkin are also good sources of calcium and other minerals.
- Include a good serving of the following plant oestrogens in your diet daily: soy products including So Good soy milk with cereals or mixed fruit as a fruit shake, tofu and silken tofu blended with fruit, golden linseeds, chick peas, lentils, mung beans, alfalfa, sunflower, pumpkin and sesame seeds and green and yellow vegetables.
- Limit your intake of fats to 30 per cent of the total calories you consume every day. For most of us this means reducing our fat intake by about a quarter. Avoid the use of lard and excessive amounts of butter and hydrogenated vegetable oil such as shortening and hard margarines. Instead, use cold pressed safflower, olive, sesame and sunflower oils. For example, use safflower oil in mayonnaise, olive oil for salads and all four oils for cooking.
- Drink plenty of liquids. Drink three to six large glasses of water daily, preferably filtered or bottled. You might like to add lemon juice to taste. Tap and mineral water can contain some calcium and magnesium. If you must drink tea and coffee use decaffeinated or, better still, herb teas or coffee substitutes. When giving up caffeine remember you may suffer headaches for a few days. Also refer to the recommendartions over the page.

- Keep the consumption of alcohol to a maximum of three to four drinks each week. Alcohol knocks most nutrients sideways and may aggravate hot flushes.
- If you smoke, try to cut down gradually as smoking can aggravate some symptoms especially hot flushes and nightsweats. Pace yourself during the day, waiting for longer periods of time between each cigarette.
- Arm yourself with nutritious snacks to eat in-between meals if you are hungry. Nuts and raisins and fresh or dried fruit are fine. If you keep your blood-sugar levels constant there is less chance of you dipping into the biscuit tin.

Coffee substitutes

There are a number of coffee substitutes you can try. If you are avoiding grains as you might have to (see Option Three), you will be restricted to dandelion coffee, instant (which is quite sweet) or dandelion root, which you grind into a granual powder and boil or put through a coffee filter – it makes a nice malted drink – or alternatively a chicory drink. There is a wider choice if you remain on grains, or when you re-introduce them to your diet. You can try Barley cup which is a very acceptable cereal-based alternative, or No Caf, available in health-food shops. You can have up to two cups of decaffeinated coffee each day, either instant or filter.

Herbal teas and tea substitutes

Redbush herbal tea lookalike is the most tea-like alternative. It comes in teabags and can be made with or without milk. Interestingly it contains a mild, natural muscle relaxant which may help alleviate tension and ease period pains if you are still menstruating. It is favoured by many of our patients and is definitely worth a try. Other suggestions are ginseng, fennel, raspberry and ginseng tea, mixed berry tea, lemon verbena and wild strawberry tea. These days most health-food shops sell single sachets so that you can 'buy and try' without being saddled with a whole box of teabags you absolutely detest.

Cold drinks

Soft drinks should be non-carbonated, sugar free, phosphate-free and decaffeinated. As the phosphorus in fizzy drinks blocks the uptake of magnesium and calcium by bone tissue, it is better if you keep fizzy drinks to a minimum. Drink plenty of still water, either bottled or filtered, with or without fruit juice and have small quantities of mineral water,

Amé, Appletise, Aqua Libra and other water- and fruit-juice-based drinks. Avoid cola drinks and other canned and bottled drinks that contain anything other than natural ingredients. Read the labels carefully before buying.

Other useful self-help tips

- Wear several layers of thin, comfortable clothing during the day so that you can peel them off should the need arise.
- Use lightweight layers of bedclothes so that you can adjust them according to your temperature. Wear cotton nightdresses instead of man-made fibres.
- Carry some cool wipes in your handbag until the flushes have abated.
- Take extra care of your hair, skin and nails. Use rich hair conditioner, good moisturising lotions for your skin and nail strengtheners.
- Do toning pelvic floor exercises once or twice a day in your spare time. Draw the vaginal muscles in and hold while you count to 10. Release them slowly. Repeat this 10 times.
- Spend time learning to relax if you have not already mastered the art. Get your partner to give you a massage if you are feeling tense, or treat yourself to one on a regular basis.
- Learn some simple yoga exercises and make some time to put them into practice each day, even if you can only manage them for 10 to 15 minutes. Remember: relaxation and rest tend to minimise flushes whereas constant activity and stress tend to make them worse.

18

OPTION TWO: A SPECIALISED PLAN FOR MODERATE SUFFERERS

As well as following the general recommendations for mild sufferers from Option One, you will need to choose specific nutrients, according to your symptoms, by referring to the following chart. You can do this initially in two ways. First, refer to the section on the Nutritional Content of Foods on pages 227–238. Choose the foods you like that contain substantial amounts of the nutrients you need. Second, take extra nutritional supplements where you feel it's appropriate (see page 118 for our recommendations).

NUTRIENTS FOR MENOPAUSAL SYMPTOMS

In conjunction with other dietary measures, plus moderate exercise and regular periods of relaxation, you will find that the following nutrients make an enormous difference to specific symptoms, as well as helping to prevent osteoporosis:

General symptoms
Concentrate on taking Novogen Red Clover, magnesium, calcium and the B vitamins.

Hot flushes
Concentrate on taking Novogen Red Clover, vitamin E, essential fatty acids and ginseng.

Anxiety attacks
Valerina, Kava Kava, B vitamins and magnesium.

Depression
Concentrate on taking St John's Wort, B vitamins, vitamins C and E and magnesium.

Lack of libido
Novogen Red Clover, magnesium, zinc, iron and B vitamins.

Heavy periods
Concentrate on eating an iron-rich diet and taking Novogen Red Clover.

Skin problems
Concentrate on taking zinc and B vitamins.

Prevention of osteoporosis
Concentrate on taking calcium, magnesium, and essential fatty acids in evening primrose oil and fish oil, and on eating a diet rich in phytoestrogens, including plenty of soy protein.

Make a note of the nutrients that you feel you need and look them up in the Nutritional Content of Foods on the following pages. From these lists you can select the foods and drinks you wish to include in your daily diet. I have suggested a one-week sample menu, which is generally high in important nutrients, to give you some ideas. You can either follow the menu exactly to get yourself started, or you can use it as a guideline and adapt it to suit your tastes and needs.

Don't eat too much red meat at the time of the menopause, as it is acknowledged that vegetarians have an easier menopause. Concentrate on eating lean poultry, fish and vegetarian protein.

Buying food

Ensure you eat plenty of salads, vegetables and fruit, no matter which option you choose, but you will have realised that many of these foods are contaminated with chemicals. Fortunately, most of the large supermarkets now stock organic produce. Although this is a little more expensive, do try to buy at least some organic produce – unless you grow your own, which makes even more sense.

The recipe section contains many vegetarian suggestions and recipes but meat and fish eaters have also been catered for. Again, because of the chemicals and hormones in meat, I would suggest you try to find a butcher who sells additive-free meat. Some supermarkets now sell it, as do the small organic farms dotted around the UK.

Vitamins and Minerals – do you lack them?

	Food sources	What they do
Vitamin B6	Meat, fish, nuts, bananas, avocados, wholegrains	Essential in the metabolism of protein and the amino acids that control mood and behaviour. Affect hormone metabolism
Vitamin B1 Thiamin	Meat, fish, nuts, wholegrains and fortified breakfast cereals	Essential in the metabolism of sugar, especially in nerves and muscles
Vitamin C Ascorbic acid	Any fresh fruits and vegetables	Involved in healing, repair of tissues and production of some hormones
Iron	Meat, wholegrains, nuts, eggs and fortified breakfast cereals	Essential to make blood-haemoglobin. Many other tissues need iron for energy reactions
Zinc	Meat, wholegrains, nuts, peas, beans, lentils	Essential for normal growth, mental function, hormone production and resistance to infection
Magnesium	Green vegetables, wholegrains, Brazil and almond nuts, many other non-junk foods	Essential for sugar and energy metabolism, needed for healthy nerves and muscles
Calcium	Milk, cheese, bread, especially white, sardines, other fish with bones, green vegetables and beans	Needed for strong teeth and bones, also for normal nerve and muscle function. Lack leads to osteoporosis – bone thinning

	Food sources	What they do
Essential Fatty Acids – Omega 3	Cod liver oil, mackerel, herring	Help to control inflammation
Fish and related oils	Salmon, rapeseed and soy bean oil	Reduce calcium losses in urine
Essential Fatty Acids – Omega 6 Evening Primrose and related oil	Sunflower, safflower and corn oils, many nuts (not peanuts) and seeds, green vegetables	Control inflammation, needed for health of nervous system, skin and blood vessels
Vitamin D	Milk, margarine, sardines, cod liver oil, eggs (and sunlight)	For the balance of calcium in bones and teeth, and for muscle strength
Vitamin E	Most nuts, seeds and vegetable oils and dark green leafy vegetables	Protect tissues from wear and tear, keep cholestrol and other fats from deteriorating inside the body
Vitamin K	Green leafy vegetables and the bacteria in our intestines	Help with blood clotting
Folic acid	All green leafy vegetables, liver and fortified cereals	Help maintain the health of the nervous system and the blood

Deficiencies

Who is at risk	Symptoms	Visible signs
Women, especially smokers, 'junk-eaters'	Depression, anxiety, insomnia, loss of responsibility	Dry/greasy facial skin, cracking at corners of mouth
Alcohol consumers, women on the pill, breast-feeding mothers, high consumers of sugar	Depression, anxiety, poor appetite, nausea, personality change	None usually! Heart, nerve and muscle problems if severe
Smokers particularly	Lethargy, depression, hypochondriasis (imagined illnesses)	Easy bruising, look for small pinpoint bruises under the tongue
Women who have heavy periods (e.g. coil users), vegetarians, especially if tea or coffee drinkers, women with recurrent thrush	Fatigue, poor energy, depression, poor digestion, sore tongue, cracking at corners of mouth	Pale complexion, brittle nails, cracking at corners of mouth
Vegetarians, especially tea and coffee drinkers, alcohol consumers, long-term users of diuretics (water pills)	Poor mental function, skin problems in general, repeated infections	Eczema, acne, greasy or dry facial skin
Women with PMS! (some 50 per cent may be lacking), long-term diuretic users, alcohol consumers	Nausea, apathy, loss of appetite, depression, mood changes, muscle cramps	Usually NONE! so easily missed; muscle spasms sometimes
Low dairy consumers, heavy drinkers, smokers, women with early menopause, lack of exercise increases the rate of bone loss-calcium in later years	Usually none until osteoporotic fracture of hip or spine. Back pain	Loss of height

Who is at risk	Symptoms	Visible signs
Those on a poor diet	None	None
Older people, diabetics, drinkers	None	None
Those on a poor diet, diabetics and drinkers. Also those with severe eczema and premenstrual breast tenderness	None	Possibly dry skin
Urban-dwelling, dark-skinned immigrants, especially young children and pregnant women, those with little sunlight exposure	Softening of the bones, poor teeth and weakness of the hip muscles	Enlarged skull, bowing of the legs and a waddling gait
Those on a very poor diet, or with serious absorption problems	None. Damage to the nervous system is severe	None
Those with a poor diet or on long-term antibiotics	Prolonged bleeding	None
Those on a poor diet, those taking anti-epileptic medication, coeliacs, and a percentage of the normal population of child-bearing women who are at increased risk of having a child with neural tube defect	Often none. Possibly depression, fatigue and poor memory	None unless anaemic

Vegetarians

If you have been eating a good vegetarian diet for some time, in theory you should by now be reaping the benefits. Vegetarians do need to pay particular attention to certain aspects of their diet, so that they do not become nutritionally deficient. Although many vegetarians and vegans take great care with their diet, there are still too many who try to exist on lettuce leaves. Apart from all the recommendations made so far, vegetarians and vegans should concentrate on making sure they have an adequate balance of proteins in their diet. No single vegetarian protein contains all the appropriate nutrients required, so it's important to combine the different types of vegetable proteins. These include nuts, seeds, peas, beans, lentils, whole-grains, brown rice, sprouted-bean and soy-bean products and are particularly important for menopausal women.

Although beans are particularly nutritious, they often cause abdominal wind. Soaking them for 24 hours before cooking them, and dehusking them, may reduce the problem.

There are many vegetarian suggestions in the body of the menus. You can use these, and you will also find a one-week suggested vegetarian menu on page 241.

NUTRITIONAL CONTENT OF FOODS

The following lists detail the foods that contain good amounts of each of the vitamins and minerals that will help combat your menopause symptoms. Read the lists through carefully to see which nutrients your favourite foods contain.

Foods containing Vitamin A – Retinol
(Micrograms per 100 g/3.5 oz)

	mcg		mcg
Skimmed milk	1	Cheddar cheese	325
Semi-skimmed milk	21	Margarine	800
Grilled herring	49	Butter	815
Whole milk	52	Lamb's liver	15,000
Porridge made with milk	56		

Foods containing Vitamin B1 – Thiamin
(Milligrams per 100 g/3.5 oz)

	mg		mg
Peaches	0.02	Oranges	0.10
Cottage cheese	0.02	Brussels sprouts	0.10
Cox's apple	0.03	Potatoes, new, boiled	0.11
Full-fat milk	0.04	Soy beans, boiled	0.12
Skimmed milk	0.04	Red peppers, raw	0.12
Semi-skimmed milk	0.04	Lentils, boiled	0.14
Cheddar cheese	0.04	Steamed salmon	0.20
Bananas	0.04	Corn	0.20
White grapes	0.04	White spaghetti, boiled	0.21
French beans	0.04	Almonds	0.24
Low-fat yogurt	0.05	White self-raising flour	0.30
Cantaloupe melon	0.05	Plaice, steamed	0.30
Tomato	0.06	Bacon, cooked	0.35
Green peppers, raw	0.07	Walnuts	0.40
Boiled egg	0.08	Wholemeal flour	0.47
Roast chicken	0.08	Lamb's kidney	0.49
Grilled cod	0.08	Brazil nuts	1.00
Haddock, steamed	0.08	Cornflakes	1.00
Roast turkey	0.09	Rice Krispies	1.00
Mackerel, cooked	0.09	Wheatgerm	2.01
Savoy cabbage, boiled	0.10		

Foods containing Vitamin B2 – Riboflavin
(Milligrams per 100 g/3.5 oz)

	mg		mg
Cabbage, boiled	0.01	Baked salmon	0.11
Potatoes, boiled	0.01	Red peppers, raw	0.15
Brown rice, boiled	0.02	Full-fat milk	0.17
Pear	0.03	Avocado	0.18
Wholemeal spaghetti, boiled	0.03	Grilled herring	0.18
		Semi-skimmed milk	0.18
White self-raising flour	0.03	Roast chicken	0.19
Orange	0.04	Roast turkey	0.21
Spinach, boiled in salted water	0.05	Cottage cheese	0.26
		Soy flour	0.31
Baked beans	0.06	Boiled prawns	0.34
Banana	0.06	Boiled egg	0.35
White bread	0.06	Topside of beef, cooked	0.35

Foods containing Vitamin B2 – Riboflavin (cont)

	mg		mg
Green peppers, raw	0.08	Leg of lamb, cooked	0.38
Lentils, boiled	0.08	Cheddar cheese	0.40
Hovis	0.09	Muesli	0.70
Soy beans, boiled	0.09	Almonds	0.75
Wholemeal bread	0.09	Cornflakes	1.50
Wholemeal flour	0.09	Rice Krispies	1.50
Peanuts	0.10		

Foods containing Vitamin B3 – Niacin
(Milligrams per 100 g/3.5 oz)

	mcg		mcg
Boiled egg	0.07	White self-raising flour	1.50
Cheddar cheese	0.07	Grilled cod	1.70
Full-fat milk	0.08	White bread	1.70
Skimmed milk	0.09	Soy flour	2.00
Semi-skimmed milk	0.09	Red peppers, raw	2.20
Cottage cheese	0.13	Almonds	3.10
Cox's apple	0.20	Grilled herring	4.00
Cabbage, boiled	0.30	Wholemeal bread	4.10
Orange	0.40	Hovis	4.20
Baked beans	0.50	Wholemeal flour	5.70
Potatoes, boiled	0.50	Muesli	6.50
Soy beans, boiled	0.50	Topside of beef, cooked	6.50
Lentils, boiled	0.60	Leg of lamb, cooked	6.60
Banana	0.70	Baked salmon	7.00
Tomato	1.00	Roast chicken	8.20
Avocado	1.10	Roast turkey	8.50
Green peppers, raw	1.10	Boiled prawns	9.50
Brown rice	1.30	Peanuts	13.80
Wholemeal spaghetti,		Cornflakes	16.00
boiled	1.30	Rice Krispies	16.00

Foods containing Vitamin B6 – Pyridoxine
(Milligrams per 100 g/3.5 oz)

	mg		mg
Carrots	0.05	Brussels sprouts	0.19
Full-fat milk	0.06	Sweetcorn, boiled	0.21
Skimmed milk	0.06	Leg of lamb, cooked	0.22
Semi-skimmed milk	0.06	Grapefruit juice	0.23
Satsumas	0.07	Roast chicken	0.26
White bread	0.07	Lentils, boiled	0.28
White rice	0.07	Banana	0.29
Cabbage, boiled	0.08	Brazil nuts	0.31
Cottage cheese	0.08	Potatoes, boiled	0.32
Cox's apple	0.08	Roast turkey	0.33
Wholemeal pasta	0.08	Grilled herring	0.33
Frozen peas	0.09	Topside of beef, cooked	0.33
Spinach, boiled	0.09	Avocado	0.36
Cheddar cheese	0.10	Grilled cod	0.38
Orange	0.10	Baked salmon	0.57
Broccoli	0.11	Soy flour	0.57
Hovis	0.11	Hazelnuts	0.59
Baked beans	0.12	Peanuts	0.59
Boiled egg	0.12	Walnuts	0.67
Red kidney beans, cooked	0.12	Muesli	1.60
Wholemeal bread	0.12	Cornflakes	1.80
Tomatoes	0.14	Rice Krispies	1.80
Almonds	0.15	Special K	2.20
Cauliflower	0.15		

Foods containing Vitamin B12
(Micrograms per 100 g/3.5 oz)

	mcg		mcg
Tempeh	0.10	Rice Krispies	2.00
Miso	0.20	Steak, lean, grilled	2.00
Quorn	0.30	Edam cheese	2.10
Full-fat milk	0.40	Eggs, whole, battery	2.40
Skimmed milk	0.40	Milk, dried, whole	2.40
Semi-skimmed milk	0.40	Milk, dried, skimmed	2.60
Marmite	0.50	Eggs, whole, free-range	2.70
Cottage cheese	0.70	Kambu seaweed	2.80
Choux buns	1.00	Squid, frozen	2.90
Eggs, boiled	1.00	Taramasalata	2.90

Foods containing Vitamin B12 (cont)

	mcg		mcg
Eggs, poached	1.00	Duck, cooked	3.00
Halibut, steamed	1.00	Turkey, dark meat	3.00
Lobster, boiled	1.00	Grapenuts	5.00
Sponge cake	1.00	Tuna in oil	5.00
Turkey, white meat	1.00	Herring, cooked	6.00
Waffles	1.00	Herring roe, fried	6.00
Cheddar cheese	1.20	Steamed salmon	6.00
Eggs, scrambled	1.20	Bovril	8.30
Squid	1.30	Mackerel, fried	10.00
Eggs, fried	1.60	Rabbit, stewed	10.00
Shrimps, boiled	1.80	Cod's roe, fried	11.00
Parmesan cheese	1.90	Pilchards canned in	
Beef, lean	2.00	tomato juice	12.00
Cod, baked	2.00	Oysters, raw	15.00
Cornflakes	2.00	Nori seaweed	27.50
Pork, cooked	2.00	Sardines in oil	28.00
Raw beef mince	2.00	Lamb's kidney, fried	79.00

Foods containing Folate/Folic acid
(Micrograms per 100 g/3.5 oz)

	mcg		mcg
Cox's apple	4.00	Orange	31.00
Leg of lamb, cooked	4.00	Baked beans	33.00
Full-fat milk	6.00	Cheddar cheese	33.00
Skimmed milk	6.00	Clementines	33.00
Semi-skimmed milk	6.00	Raspberries	33.00
Porridge with		Satsumas	33.00
semi-skimmed milk	7.00	Blackberries	34.00
Turnip, baked	8.00	Rye crispbread	35.00
Sweet potato, boiled	8.00	Potato, baked in skin	36.00
Cucumber	9.00	Radish	38.00
Grilled herring	10.00	Boiled egg	39.00
Roast chicken	10.00	Hovis	39.00
Avocado	11.00	Wholemeal bread	39.00
Grilled cod	12.00	Red kidney beans, boiled	42.00
Banana	14.00	Potato, baked	44.00
Roast turkey	15.00	Frozen peas	47.00
Carrots	17.00	Almonds	48.00
Sweet potato	17.00	Parsnips, boiled	48.00

Foods containing Folate/Folic acid (cont)

	mcg		mcg
Tomatoes	17.00	Cauliflower	51.00
Topside of beef, cooked	17.00	Green beans, boiled	57.00
Swede, boiled	18.00	Broccoli	64.00
Strawberries	20.00	Walnuts	66.00
Brazil nuts	21.00	Artichoke	68.00
Red peppers, raw	21.00	Hazelnuts	72.00
Green peppers, raw	23.00	Spinach, boiled	90.00
Rye bread	24.00	Brussels sprouts	110.00
Dates, fresh	25.00	Peanuts	110.00
New potatoes, boiled	25.00	Muesli	140.00
Grapefruit	26.00	Sweetcorn, boiled	150.00
Oatcakes	26.00	Asparagus	155.00
Cottage cheese	27.00	Chickpeas	180.00
Baked salmon	29.00	Lamb's liver, fried	240.00
Cabbage, boiled	29.00	Cornflakes	250.00
Onions, boiled	29.00	Rice Krispies	250.00
White bread	29.00	Calf's liver, fried	320.00

Foods containing Vitamin C

(Milligrams per 100 g/3.5 oz)

	mg		mg
Full-fat milk	1.00	Melon	17.00
Skimmed milk	1.00	Tomatoes	17.00
Semi-skimmed milk	1.00	Cabbage, boiled	20.00
Red kidney beans	1.00	Canteloupe melon	26.00
Carrots	2.00	Cauliflower	27.00
Cucumber	2.00	Satsumas	27.00
Muesli with dried fruit	2.00	Peach	31.00
Apricots, raw	6.00	Raspberries	32.00
Avocado	6.00	Bran flakes	35.00
Pear	6.00	Grapefruit	36.00
Potato, boiled	6.00	Mangoes	37.00
Spinach, boiled	8.00	Nectarine	37.00
Cox's apple	9.00	Kumquats	39.00
Turnip	10.00	Broccoli	44.00
Banana	11.00	Lychees	45.00
Frozen peas	12.00	Unsweetened apple juice	49.00
Lamb's liver, fried	12.00	Orange	54.00
Pineapple	12.00	Kiwi fruit	59.00
Dried skimmed milk	13.00	Brussels sprouts	60.00
Gooseberries	14.00	Strawberries	77.00
Raw dates	14.00	Blackcurrants	115.00

Foods containing Vitamin D
(Micrograms per 100 g/3.5 oz)

	mcg		mcg
Skimmed milk	0.01	Cornflakes	2.80
Whole milk	0.03	Rice Krispies	2.80
Fromage frais	0.05	Kellogg's Start	4.20
Cheddar cheese	0.26	Margarine	8.00

Foods containing Vitamin E
(Milligrams per 100 g/3.5 oz)

	mg		mg
Semi-skimmed milk	0.03	Unsweetened orange juice	0.68
Boiled potatoes	0.06	Leeks	0.78
Cucumber	0.07	Sweetcorn, boiled	0.88
Cottage cheese	0.08	Brussels sprouts	0.90
Full-fat milk	0.09	Broccoli	1.10
Cabbage, boiled	0.10	Boiled egg	1.11
Leg of lamb, cooked	0.10	Tomato	1.22
Cauliflower	0.11	Watercress	1.46
Roast chicken	0.11	Parsley	1.70
Frozen peas	0.18	Spinach, boiled	1.71
Red kidney beans, cooked	0.20	Olives	1.99
Wholemeal bread	0.20	Butter	2.00
Orange	0.24	Onions, dried raw	2.69
Topside of beef, cooked	0.26	Mushrooms, fried in corn	
Banana	0.27	oil	2.84
Brown rice, boiled	0.30	Avocado	3.20
Grilled herring	0.30	Muesli	3.20
Lamb's liver, fried	0.32	Walnuts	3.85
Baked beans	0.36	Peanut butter	4.99
Cornflakes	0.40	Olive oil	5.10
Pear	0.50	Sweet potato, baked	5.96
Cheddar cheese	0.53	Brazil nuts	7.18
Carrots	0.56	Peanuts	10.09
Lettuce	0.57	Pine nuts	13.65
Cox's apple	0.59	Rapeseed oil	18.40
Grilled cod	0.59	Almonds	23.96
Rice Krispies	0.60	Hazelnuts	24.98
Plums	0.61	Sunflower oil	48.70

Foods containing Calcium
(Milligrams per 100 g/3.5 oz)

	mg		mg
Cox's apple	4.00	Orange	47.00
Brown rice, boiled	4.00	Baked beans	48.00
Potatoes, boiled	5.00	Wholemeal bread	54.00
Banana	6.00	Boiled egg	57.00
Topside of beef, cooked	6.00	Peanuts	60.00
White pasta, boiled	7.00	Cottage cheese	73.00
Tomato	7.00	Soy beans, boiled	83.00
White spaghetti, boiled	7.00	White bread	100.00
Leg of lamb, cooked	8.00	Full-fat milk	115.00
Red peppers, raw	8.00	Hovis	120.00
Roast chicken	9.00	Muesli	120.00
Roast turkey	9.00	Skimmed milk	120.00
Avocado	11.00	Semi-skimmed milk	120.00
Pear	11.00	Prawns, boiled	150.00
Butter	15.00	Spinach, boiled	150.00
Cornflakes	15.00	Brazil nuts	170.00
White rice, boiled	18.00	Yogurt, low-fat, natural	190.00
Grilled cod	22.00	Soy flour	210.00
Lentils, boiled	22.00	Almonds	240.00
Baked salmon	29.00	White self-raising flour	450.00
Green peppers, raw	30.00	Sardines	550.00
Young carrots	30.00	Sprats, fried	710.00
Grilled herring	33.00	Cheddar cheese	720.00
Wholemeal flour	38.00	Whitebait, fried	860.00
Turnips, baked	45.00		

Foods containing Chromium
(Milligrams per 100 g/3.5 oz)

	mcg		mcg
Egg yolk	183.00	Hard cheese	56.00
Molasses	121.00	Liver	55.00
Brewer's yeast	117.00	Fruit juices	47.00
Beef	57.00	Wholemeal bread	42.00

Foods containing Iron
(Milligrams per 100 g/3.5 oz)

	mg		mg
Semi-skimmed milk	0.05	Boiled prawns	1.10
Skimmed milk	0.06	Green peppers, raw	1.20
Full-fat milk	0.06	Baked beans	1.40
Cottage cheese	0.10	Wholemeal spaghetti,	
Orange	0.10	boiled	1.40
Cox's apple	0.20	White bread	1.60
Pear	0.20	Spinach, boiled	1.70
White rice	0.20	Boiled egg	1.90
Banana	0.30	White self-raising flour	2.00
Cabbage, boiled	0.30	Brazil nuts	2.50
Cheddar cheese	0.30	Peanuts	2.50
Avocado	0.40	Leg of lamb, cooked	2.70
Grilled cod	0.40	Wholemeal bread	2.70
Potatoes, boiled	0.40	Topside of beef, cooked	2.80
Young carrots, boiled	0.40	Almonds	3.00
Brown rice, boiled	0.50	Soy beans, boiled	3.00
Tomato	0.50	Lentils, boiled	3.50
White pasta, boiled	0.50	Hovis	3.70
Baked salmon	0.80	Wholemeal flour	3.90
Roast chicken	0.80	Muesli	5.60
Roast turkey	0.90	Cornflakes	6.70
Grilled herring	1.00	Rice Krispies	6.70
Red peppers, raw	1.00	Soy flour	6.90

Foods containing Magnesium
(Milligrams per 100 g/3.5 oz)

	mg		mg
Butter	2.00	Grilled cod	26.00
Cox's apple	6.00	Roast turkey	27.00
Turnip, baked	6.00	Leg of lamb, cooked	28.00
Young carrots	6.00	Baked salmon	29.00
Tomato	7.00	Baked beans	31.00
Cottage cheese	9.00	Spinach, boiled	31.00
Orange	10.00	Grilled herring	32.00
Full-fat milk	11.00	Banana	34.00
White rice, boiled	11.00	Lentils, boiled	34.00
Semi-skimmed milk	11.00	Boiled prawns	42.00
Skimmed milk	12.00	Wholemeal spaghetti,	
Boiled egg	12.00	boiled	42.00
Cornflakes	14.00	Brown rice, boiled	43.00
Potatoes, boiled	14.00	Hovis	56.00
Red peppers, raw	14.00	Soy beans, boiled	63.00
White pasta	15.00	Wholemeal bread	76.00
White self-raising flour	20.00	Muesli	85.00
Green peppers, raw	24.00	Wholemeal flour	120.00
Roast chicken	24.00	Peanuts	210.00
Topside of beef, cooked	24.00	Soy flour	240.00
White bread	24.00	Almonds	270.00
Avocado	25.00	Brazil nuts	410.00
Cheddar cheese	25.00		

Foods containing Selenium
(Micrograms per 100 g/3.5 oz)

	mcg		mcg
Full-fat milk	1.00	White rice	4.00
Semi-skimmed milk	1.00	White self-raising flour	4.00
Skimmed milk	1.00	Soy beans, boiled	5.00
Baked beans	2.00	Boiled egg	11.00
Cornflakes	2.00	Cheddar cheese	12.00
Orange	2.00	White bread	28.00
Peanuts	3.00	Wholemeal bread	35.00
Almonds	4.00	Lentils, boiled	40.00
Cottage cheese	4.00	Wholemeal flour	53.00

Foods containing Zinc
(Milligrams per 100 g/3.5 oz)

	mg		mg
Butter	0.10	White self-raising flour	0.60
Pear	0.10	Brown rice	0.70
Orange	0.10	White rice	0.70
Red peppers, raw	0.10	Soy beans, boiled	0.90
Banana	0.20	Wholemeal spaghetti, boiled	1.10
Young carrots	0.20		
Cornflakes	0.30	Boiled egg	1.30
Potatoes, boiled	0.30	Lentils, boiled	1.40
Avocado	0.40	Roast chicken	1.50
Full-fat milk	0.40	Boiled prawns	1.60
Skimmed milk	0.40	Wholemeal bread	1.80
Green peppers, raw	0.40	Hovis	2.10
Semi-skimmed milk	0.40	Cheddar cheese	2.30
Baked beans	0.50	Roast turkey	2.40
Grilled cod	0.50	Muesli	2.50
Grilled herring	0.50	Wholemeal flour	2.90
White pasta	0.50	Almonds	3.20
Tomatoes	0.50	Peanuts	3.50
Cottage cheese	0.60	Brazil nuts	4.20
Spinach, boiled	0.60	Leg of lamb, cooked	5.30
White bread	0.60	Topside of beef, cooked	5.50

Foods containing Essential fatty acids

Exact amounts of these fats are hard to quantify. Good sources for the two families of essential fatty acids are given.

Omega 6 Series Essential Fatty Acids
Sunflower oil
Rapeseed oil
Corn oil
Almonds
Walnuts
Brazil nuts
Sunflower seeds
Soy products including tofu

Omega 3 Series Essential Fatty Acids
Mackerel
Herring } fresh cooked or smoked/pickled
Salmon
Walnuts and walnut oil
Rapeseed oil
Soy products and soy oil

ONE-WEEK SAMPLE MENUS

Dishes marked * are given in the recipe section.

DAY ONE

Breakfast
Porridge made with So Good soy
    milk
Handful of almonds
Banana, chopped
Nutritea Rooibos Gold tea

Lunch
Mackerel in tomato sauce
Green salad with a handful of
    pumpkin and sunflower seeds
Apple

Dinner
Nutty tofu risotto*
Sautéed broccoli and carrots

Dessert
Rhubarb crumble* with Soya
    Dream or soy yogurt

DAY TWO

Breakfast
Cornflakes with So Good soy milk
Handful of pumpkin and sun-
 flower seeds
Glass of freshly squeezed orange
 juice

Lunch
Watercress soup*
Rye bread or oatcakes

Small portion of cheese
Banana

Dinner
Chicken and leek sauté*
Broccoli
Potatoes
Carrots

Dessert
Lime and coconut pudding*

DAY THREE

Breakfast
2 slices wholemeal toast or 4
 oatcakes
2 boiled eggs
Glass of apple juice

Lunch
Sardine pâté*
Green salad
Rye bread or oatcakes

Orange

Dinner
Poached cod with parsley sauce
New potatoes
Spinach
Carrots

Dessert
Mango Delight*

DAY FOUR

Breakfast
Jordan's Organic Crunchy Oat
 with So Good soy milk
Banana, chopped
Nutritea Rooibos Gold tea

Lunch
Jacket potato with hoummus
Alfalfa and cress salad*
Pear

Dinner
Chicken fricassée*
Sautéed potatoes
Courgettes
Carrots
Broccoli

Dessert
Stewed apple with cinnamon
 and ginger
Soy yogurt or So Good soy milk
 custard

DAY FIVE

Breakfast
2 slices of rye bread
2 poached eggs
Glass of freshly squeezed orange
  juice

Lunch
Cottage cheese fruit salad*
Rye crispbread or oatcakes
Soy yogurt

Dinner
Salmon steak, grilled
New potatoes
Mangetout
Ratatouille

Dessert
Sweet cherry batter
  pudding*

DAY SIX

Breakfast
Oats soaked in cold So Good
  soy milk
Handful of pumpkin and sun-
  flower seeds
Apple, chopped
Maple syrup to sweeten
Nutritea Rooibos Gold tea

Lunch
Tuna mixed with cottage cheese
Green salad
Oatcakes or French bread

Handful of almonds and pecan
  nuts
Apple

Dinner
Lemony cod and spinach bake*
New potatoes
Sweetcorn
Courgettes

Dessert
Fresh fruit salad with Soya
  Dream

DAY SEVEN

Breakfast
Cornflakes with So Good soy milk
Banana, chopped
Handful of pecans and almonds
Nutritea Rooibos Gold tea

Lunch
Apple and fennel soup*
Rye bread or French stick

small piece of goat's cheese
Pear

Dinner
Tofu stir fry
Rice noodles or rice

Dessert
Ricotta and almond pots*

ONE-WEEK SAMPLE MENUS
FOR VEGETARIANS

Dishes marked * are given in the recipe section.

DAY ONE

Breakfast
Jordan's Organic Crunchy Oat
  with So Good soy milk
Pear
Nutritea Rooibos Gold tea

Lunch
Oatcakes or wholemeal bread
  with peanut or almond butter
Carrot and cashew nut salad

Soy yogurt

Dinner
Cajun tofu* with brown rice

Dessert
Almond and raisin cheesecake
  bake*

DAY TWO

Breakfast
Rice Krispies with So Good soy
  milk
Pecan and almonds
Banana, chopped
Glass of apple juice

Lunch
2 slices of rye bread with hoummus
Alfalfa and cress salad

Pear

Dinner
Oat and almond bake*
Green salad

Dessert
Lime and coconut pudding*

DAY THREE

Breakfast
Jordan's Organic Muesli with So
  Good soy milk
Banana, chopped
Nutritea Rooibos Gold tea

Lunch
Avocado pear with cottage
  cheese

Pumpkin and sunflower seeds
2 oatcakes
Soy yogurt

Dinner
Tofu loaf*
Green salad

DAY FOUR

Breakfast
Pancakes made with wholemeal
    flour or rice/corn flour
Mixed summer berries
Soy yogurt
Glass of apple juice

Lunch
Sweet potato and chickpea soup*
Rye bread or oatcakes

Sesame seed bar

Dinner
Cheese and courgette kebabs*
Brown rice
Green salad

Dessert
Rhubarb oat crumble with Soya
    Dream

DAY FIVE

Breakfast
Oats soaked in cold soy milk
Dried apricots
Pecans and almonds
Glass of freshly squeezed orange
    juice

Lunch
Jacket potato with hommus

Green salad
Banana

Dinner
Vegetable quiche*
Carrot and peanut salad*

Dessert
Soy yogurt

DAY SIX

Breakfast
Fresh fruit salad (kiwi, banana,
    melon)
Natural bio or soy yogurt
Pumpkin and sunflower seeds

Lunch
Spinach and broccoli soup with
    tarragon*
Rye bread or French bread

Small portion of goat's cheese
Apple

Dinner
Sesame tofu
Rice noodles

Dessert
Burgen bread and butter
    pudding* with Soya Dream
    or soy yogurt

DAY SEVEN

Breakfast
Rice cakes or oatcakes with
  mashed banana and pure fruit
  spread
Pecans and almonds
Nutritea Rooibos Gold tea

Lunch
Jacket potato with guacamole
  and hoummus

Carrot and cashew nut salad
Fruit and nut bar

Dinner
Lentil bolognaise*
Green salad

Dessert
Mango Delight*

Easy-option lunches (not avoiding grains)

Sardines on toast
Peanut butter sandwich and fruit salad
French stick with mackerel and salad
Cheese sandwich and mixed salad
Raw vegetables with pitta bread and hoummus
Beans on toast and salad
Jacket potato with cheese or beans and salad
Mixed bean salad
Turkey salad sandwich
Stir-fry vegetables and rice
Soup and a salad
Omelette and salad
Fruit and nut salad and live yoghurt
Hoummus and alfalfa sandwich with mixed salad
Cheese omelette with salad and alfalfa sprouts
Fruit, nut and sunflower seed with soy or natural yogurt
Jacket potato with mixed beans
Cottage cheese mixed with tahini and served with raw vegetables

Easy-option dinners (not avoiding grains)

Broccoli and cauliflower cheese with jacket potato
Grilled mackerel and salad
Pasta with tomato sauce, fresh herbs, pine kernels and Parmesan cheese
Grilled lamb or pork chops with vegetables
Fresh grilled sardines and salad
Stir-fry Quorn and vegetables with rice
Kangaroo steak, chips and salad
Stir-fry vegetables and almonds with noodles
Stir-fry vegetables with prawns and rice
Hard-boiled egg and grated cheese salad
Mixed bean salad with wholemeal pitta bread
Tofu burgers and salad
Mackerel coated with rolled oats and grilled with green vegetables and salad
Stir-fry tofu and vegetables with rice
Lentil bolognaise*
Tofu risotto*
Mixed bean salad with hoummus and pitta bread
Tofu kebabs with rice and salad

Snack list

Ryvita and peanut butter or low-sugar jam
Fresh fruit, nuts and seeds
Nuts and raisins
Yogurt (live or soy)
Fruit
Jordans' oat and nut fruesli bars
Dried fruit bars like Granovita
La Fruit – dried fruit cubes
Raw vegetables and dips like hoummus or taramasalata
Pitta bread
Pasta or bean salad
Phyto-rich muesli with So Good soy milk or soy yogurt
Jordan's organic crunchy oat cereal with So Good soy milk
Oatcakes with tahini and pure fruit spread
Slice of phyto fruit loaf
Soy and linseed bread sandwich

Beverage list

Hot
Nutritea Rooibos Gold Tea
Barley cup
Dandelion coffee (instant or root)
Fennel tea
Ginseng tea
Raspberry and ginseng tea
Other herbal teas and coffee substitutes
No Caf cereal coffee substitute
Lemon and ginger tea
Fennel tea
Barley cup

No more than two cups of decaffeinated drinks per day.

Cold
Small amount of carbonated water
Fruit juice diluted to taste
Small amounts of Appletise or similar drinks
Mixed fruit cocktails
Amé
Aqua Libra
Fruit juice
Mineral water
Ginger cordial

Only very small amounts of alcohol as it may aggravate flushing and impedes the absorption of most nutrients.

19
OPTION THREE: A TAILOR-MADE PROGRAMME FOR SEVERE SUFFERERS

Once you have chosen your programme you will need to follow it. That may sound a bit obvious, but it does take time to adjust to a new way of eating. Changing the habits of a lifetime is not always easy and initially you will need a good deal of discipline and will-power. If you choose Option Three, presumably it will be because you are suffering severely. In my experience of dealing with severe sufferers, their very suffering is enough to motivate them initially. When the symptoms get bad, most people are willing to make short-term sacrifices. It is the first month that is usually the most difficult. Not only do you have to discipline yourself to follow a new and different regime while you are still feeling rough, but you may also encounter some withdrawal symptoms when you eliminate foods and drinks that have become a habit.

Withdrawal symptoms may occur during the first few days on the programme and can sometimes last for as long as two weeks. Although they don't always happen, it's worth remembering that they are very common. Depriving the body of things it has grown used to sometimes causes it to 'bite back'. It may seem strange that this should occur as a result of dietary changes, but it's similar to the mechanism of withdrawing from drugs or alcohol. Because of this it's best to start your programme when you have a few quiet days or, better still, a quiet week. If you experience headaches or extra nervous tension or fatigue, you will be able to relax or lie quietly in a cool, darkened room.

Giving up tea and coffee, for example, may trigger off a number of changes in your body. These may make you feel tired or uptight, anxious or on edge. Headaches may occur and, more often, the desire to eat seems to persist. You will be pleased to hear that all this settles down within days, certainly within a few weeks. Once you have passed through this stage, if it happens to you at all, life becomes much easier and before long you will notice new habit patterns forming. For example, you may even lose your desire for salty food and regular cups of strong coffee.

It is certainly worth persevering for there is light at the end of the tunnel. Our research proves this very strongly. We analysed the results of a group of 50 menopausal women who went through our four-month nutritional programme, making the recommended dietary changes and taking regular weight-bearing exercise. They also took the vitamin and mineral supplement Gynovite Plus. This particular nutritional supplement contains substantial quantities of the essential vitamins and minerals, particularly calcium and magnesium. The results of the analysis showed that just over 80 per cent of the women felt that their symptoms had been completely controlled or much improved by the nutritional programme. Only one woman in the sample felt that her symptoms had not been helped at all.

If I haven't put you off – let's get down to it! First, prepare a personal nutritional programme (see page 215). Read through the Nutritional Content of Food lists starting on page 227 and, with the exception of any food or drink you decide to steer clear of, you can choose the foods and drinks you like, knowing they are rich in important nutrients. As your symptoms are severe it would probably be a good idea initially to incorporate foods from all the nutrient lists. Then refer again to the chapters on supplement recommendations, exercise and stress and relaxation on pages 150, 165, 178. Add on to your personal chart the supplements you decide to take and make a note of the exercise you intend to carry out each week. Note the actual exercise schedule as well as the *type* of exercise.

Sample menus and recipes are laid out for you to follow for one week. There are also simple alternatives in case you do not feel like cooking or have a hectic lifestyle. Many of the easy options are quick to prepare and are portable if you are eating lunch at work or away from home. If you are careful, you should be able to eat your way around most restaurant menus, but it may take you a while to get used to doing so.

SENSITIVITY TO GRAINS

There is evidence to show that many menopausal symptoms may be related to food sensitivity. Research suggests that a significant percentage of the population produce antibodies to some foods. In our experience, this may be only a temporary state of affairs that occurs when we are not in very good nutritional shape. Finding the right kind of diet for your body will help to overcome your symptoms. It's therefore worth avoiding certain groups of foods temporarily if you suffer with the symptoms in this section. Try to follow the recommendations closely: you will reap the benefit.

The most common sensitivity is to wholewheat and grains, and many symptoms such as irritability, abdominal bloating, constipation, diarrhoea, excessive wind, irritable bowel, fatigue and depression can be aggravated by eating foods containing them. Certain people react to wheat, oats, barley and rye and all foods made from or containing them. They are therefore better off avoiding them altogether initially until the symptoms are under control. It sounds a bit drastic, but there are many alternative foods that can be used instead.

Bread

Both chemists and health-food shops usually have some stocks of alternative grain products; in our experience, chemists are usually the most reasonably priced. They will usually hold a stock of products for people with gluten allergy.

Look out for some of the following products:

- EnerG white or brown rice bread (which toasts nicely)
- Glutafin wheat-free bread and rolls
- Glutano make a flat bread like pumpernickel which is made from rice and corn. It is lovely as a base for open sandwiches.
- Barkat white and brown rice bread which can be gently warmed or toasted for best results
- Dr Scharr wheat- and gluten-free bread rolls and baguettes
- Pleni day gluten-free part baked rolls
- Orgran corn crispbreads, plain or paprika flavoured
- There are also a number of very acceptable crackers. Glutano Crackers are my favourite, but Orgran and Glutafin make rice corn and rice crackers, all of which are available from health-food shops.
- Rice cakes (now available as squares) are also widely available in health-food shops and supermarkets.

Home-made bread
Although I have not been very successful in making bread with alternative flours, some of our patients have successfully experimented. Recipes for potato and rice bread and for buckwheat and rice bread are on pages 300–301. A new multi-purpose gluten-free flour from Dove's

Farm is excellent for making bread and scones. Delicious tried and tested recipes can be found starting on page 300.

Pasta

Although you will need to avoid pasta made with wheat, there are many reasonable alternatives. Most of these are available from health-food shops, the Chinese supermarket or the pharmacist.

Orgran produce a range of pasta made from alternative grains which is very popular with our patients.

Glutafin have a range of pasta which is sometimes available in health-food shops, and can also be ordered from the chemist.

Mrs Leeper makes corn- and rice-based alternatives to spaghetti and lasagne which the whole family can enjoy.

Rice noodles are available in a wide variety from Chinese supermarkets. There are wide, flat rice noodles that resemble tagliatelli, spaghetti-like noodles, and the very skinny variety that only need soaking in a covered pan in boiling water for a few minutes. You will probably find that these are cheaper than the alternative pastas available from health-food shops and chemists.

Breakfast cereal

Any rice or corn cereals will be fine, even the ordinary Rice Krispies and cornflakes from the supermarket, or the health-food shop equivalent. Add some chopped fruit and crumbled nuts, perhaps a few seeds and a little dried fruit to make it a bit more wholesome. There are some alternative mueslis available, but they are usually very expensive for only a small packet.

Home-baked foods

If you enjoy cooking there are plenty of very acceptable biscuits, cakes, pastries, sponges and pancakes you can make using alternative flours. If you have never used any of these before it may take you time to find the consistency you like. Dove's Farm have brought out a new multi-purpose gluten-free flour mix. It is ideal for making cakes, biscuits and bread and is very simple to use.

Sponge
Brown rice flour is probably the best for making sponge. Make it up to the recipe weight by mixing it with a some ground almond and a raising

agent (cream of tartar and bicarbonate of soda or baking powder). Soy flour is also good (if combined with brown rice or cornflour) because it tops up your daily phytoestrogen intake. Experiment with Dove's Farm gluten-free flour. It is a versatile mix for making light cakes and sponges and can be used in more conventional recipes. Terence Stamp all-purpose wheat-free flour is a mixture of barley, rice, millet and maize and works well in cookies, cakes, biscuits and scones.

Raising agents
As baking powder contains wheat, you will need to use an alternative. Either use a combination of one part of bicarbonate of soda to two parts of cream of tartar, or use Glutafin wheat-free baking powder.

Savoury pancakes
These can be made with pure buckwheat flour. Buckwheat is part of the rhubarb family, and the flour tends to be quite heavy, but it can be mixed with a little rice flour, which is light.

Sweet pancakes
These are best made with a combination of brown rice flour or ground rice (purchased from a health-food shop or Chinese supermarket) and cornflour. Use half cornflour and half rice flour to replace the normal quantity of flour in a recipe.

Breadcrumbs or batter
A crisp coating for fish or meat can be made with maize meal, sold in health-food shops. Coat the fish or meat with meal, then with beaten egg and again with meal. You can then bake, grill or even fry the food which should emerge with a crispy coat.

Pizza base
You can make a reasonable pizza base with rice, corn and gram (chickpea) flour. Use 225g (8 oz) flour, 2 tablespoons oil, and sufficient water to make a dough. Roll straight onto the baking tray and bake blind before using a topping of your choice. You can make an excellent pizza base with Dove's Farm gluten-free flour mix. For the recipe, see page 286.

Biscuits
There are varieties of biscuits that you can make using brown rice flour or ground rice and ground nuts or coconut. If you make plain biscuits you can flavour them with lemon or ginger. Our recipes for almond macaroons and coconut biscuits are very acceptable and at the same

time more nutritious than the average biscuit as they are full of eggs and nuts. Make some and keep them in the freezer.

Other flours

There are many other flours you can use in your cooking. Gram flour made from chickpeas, potato flour, soy flour, tapioca flour and millet flour are all good examples. Glutafin make flour mixes for bread, pastry and cakes, as do TruFree, and these are available in some health-food shops.

Shop-bought baked goods

Acceptable cakes and biscuits can now be purchased in health-food shops and ordered from most chemists' shops. Glutafin have a range of biscuits, including digestives, and Rite-Diet have a range of biscuits and cakes. The coconut biscuits are the least sweet and the banana or lemon cakes are also worth trying, as are Granny Ann protein biscuits. Dr Scharr and Plenî day cakes and biscuits are available from selected health-food shops. Lifestyle products manufacture gluten- and wheat-free bread, rolls, cakes and savouries and deliver them freshly baked to your door! Dove's Farm produce gluten free lemon cookies which are delicious!

Snacks

It's nice to have something to crunch on when you are avoiding wheat. There are lots of corn products available, but do remember to read the labels as some have added wheat in the form of rusk and flour. Try corn chips (Nachips), crisps and wafers and look in the Mexican section of the supermarket.

ASSESSING FOR GRAIN SENSITIVITY

You will need to become a nutritional detective by doing the following:

- Stop eating all the grains mentioned above (wheat, oats, barley, rye) for at least four, preferably six, weeks. You can eat one slice of French bread made with French flour each day if you are desperate! This may seem strange, as refined bread is nowhere near as nutritious as wholemeal. However, during the refining process most of the grain has been removed, so the degree of aggravation caused by this is far less than by a wholegrain loaf. It's better to manage on rice cakes or Glutafin crackers.

- After four or six weeks, or longer, when you feel that your symptoms have diminished, introduce the various grains one-by-one back into your diet. Begin just after your period, so that you don't confuse any reaction with menopausal symptoms. Choose one grain, like rye in the form of Ryvita. Introduce this into your diet and eat it for several days. If you have no reaction after five days, choose another grain and repeat the process. *Do not mix the grains* initially because if you do get a reaction you won't know exactly what you have reacted to! Continue to do this with all the grains, providing you don't have reactions to any one of them. Try wheat last, as this grain causes most problems.
- Once you get used to using the alternatives you shouldn't find the diet difficult to maintain. If you are going to avoid certain groups of foods for any length of time, it's important to arm yourself with all the alternative foods you can muster. It's not a weight-loss diet (although you may lose weight on it if you are overweight) and you can literally eat as much as you like of the foods on your list. Never allow yourself to get hungry and never miss a meal. It's important to eat a steady flow of good nutrients to allow your hormone- and brain-chemical metabolism to function at its best.

What to do if you have a reaction

The reactions may include diarrhoea or constipation, excessive wind, abdominal bloating, headaches, weight-gain, fatigue, confusion, depression, mouth ulcers, skin rash, irritability and palpitations.

1 Once you have established what you have reacted to, make a note of it and avoid eating this food at all for the moment. This doesn't mean that you won't ever be able to eat this food again but it's best avoided for now.
2 Wait until your body has settled down again and then try another grain.

Foods containing grains

It's surprising how many foods contain grains. Before I began 'label-reading' I would never have believed the extent to which grains are used. It's a good exercise to go around the supermarket reading labels on packets to get an idea of this for yourself. Sometimes labels aren't as explicit as they might be and they just contain the words 'edible starch'. Regard this with suspicion if you are on a grain-free diet. The labelling of food in health-food shops is usually more reliable and precise.

Wheat

The most obvious foods containing wheat are bread, biscuits, cakes, pasta, cereals, pastries and flour made from wheat, etc., but wheat is often present in prepared sauces, soups and processed foods in general, including sausages. Gluten-free products are not particularly recommended on a wheat-free diet, as some of them still contain wheat. Wheat is also disguised as modified starch, rusk, cereal filler and builders.

Oats

Porridge, oat cookies, oatcakes, flapjacks and oat flakes.

Rye

Rye bread (which may also contain wheat), Ryvita and pumpernickel.

Barley

Often found in packet or tinned soups and stews, and in barley beverages. There are many lovely recipe books available with lots of ideas. These are listed in the recommended reading section on page 322. I have also prepared some sample menus to give you an idea of the possible scope. There are also a few guideline recipes included in the recipe section on page 263.

ONE-WEEK GRAIN-FREE SAMPLE MENUS
WHEAT, OATS, BARLEY AND RYE FREE

Dishes marked * are given in the recipe section. Most recipes are marked WOBR.

DAY ONE

Breakfast
Rice Krispies with banana and
    So Good soy milk
Sunflower seeds and pecan nuts
1 tbsp golden linseeds
Glass of freshly squeezed orange
    juice

Lunch
Apple and fennel soup*

Barkat rice bread, toasted
Small portion of cheese
Apple

Dinner
Stir-fry tofu and vegetable with
    brown rice

Dessert
Frozen raspberry cheesecake*

DAY TWO

Breakfast
Rice porridge with maple syrup
Puréed apple
Pecan nuts
Nutritea Rooibos Gold tea

Lunch
Cottage cheese fruit salad
Pecans and almonds

2 rice cakes with almond butter
Pear

Dinner
Lemony cod and spinach bake*
New potatoes
Carrots
Petits pois

Dessert
Rice and almond brûlée*

DAY THREE

Breakfast
2 boiled eggs
2 rice cakes with soy spread
2 rice cakes with pure fruit spread
Glass of pineapple juice

Lunch
Jacket potato with tuna

Pineapple and watercress salad*
Banana

Dinner
Wheat-free pizza*
Alfalfa and cress*

Dessert
Crème caramel

DAY FOUR

Breakfast
Phyto-rich muesli with So Good
    soy milk
Spoonful of soy yogurt
Banana
Nutritea Rooibos Gold tea

Lunch
4 rice cakes with hoummus

Ginger, carrot and nut salad*
Fresh mango with cinnamon and
    ginger

Dinner
Oat and almond bake*
Sautéed potatoes
Courgettes
Carrots

DAY FIVE

Breakfast
2-egg omelette with mushrooms
  and cheese
Barkat rice bread toasted with
  pure fruit spread
Glass of freshly squeezed orange
  juice

Lunch
Sardine pâté*
Green salad

4 rice cakes
Banana

Dinner
Tofu kebabs with stir-fried vegetables and brown rice

Dessert
Almond and raisin cheesecake
  bake* with Soya Dream

DAY SIX

Breakfast
Cornflakes with So Good soy
  milk
1 tbsp golden linseeds
Pecan nuts and pumpkin seeds
2 rice cakes with organic honey
Nutritea Rooibos Gold tea

Lunch
Sweet potato and chickpea
  soup*

Barkat rice bread, toasted
Fresh fruit salad with soy yogurt

Dinner
Tofu loaf*
Carrot and cashew nuts salad*

Dessert
Baked custard* with mixed
  summer berries

DAY SEVEN

Breakfast
Fresh fruit salad (mango, kiwi,
  melon, banana)
Soy or bio yogurt
Pecans and almonds
2 rice cakes with organic honey
Nutritea Rooibos Gold tea

Lunch
Tinned mackerel in tomato sauce

Barkat rice bread, toasted
Slice of lemon and almond cake*

Dinner
Tofu, bean and herb stir fry*
  with rice noodles

Dessert
Honey cake* with Soya Dream

Easy-option lunches (wheat, oats, barley and rye free)

Raw vegetables and dips e.g. hoummus, taramasalata
Jacket potato with cheese and salad
Tinned mackerel and salad
Cold meat and salad
Beans on alternative toast
Stir-fry vegetables and rice
Soup and salad
Omelette and salad
Rice salad with nuts
Fruit and nut salad with live yogurt
Mixed bean salad
Stir fry tofu and vegetables with rice
Cottage cheese with mixed nuts and sunflower seeds
Cottage cheese with tuna and fresh pineapple
Tofu burgers with salad
Phyto-rich muesli with So Good soy milk

Easy-option dinners (wheat, oats, barley and rye free)

Grilled mackerel with salad
Corn pasta with tomato sauce, pine kernels and fresh herbs
Grilled lamb or pork chops with vegetables
Grilled fresh sardines with salad
Stir-fry Quorn and vegetables with rice
Stir-fry vegetables and almonds with rice noodles
Stir-fry prawns and vegetables with rice
Hard-boiled egg and grated cheese salad
Greek salad with pine nuts
Steak, chips and salad
Mixed bean salad with rice salad
Prepared Quorn and sweetcorn escalopes (frozen) with vegetables
Salmon with new potatoes and salad
Broccoli and cauliflower cheese (made with cornflour) and jacket
  potato
Grilled gammon and pineapple and vegetables
Rice pasta with tomato sauce and fresh vegetables
Stir fry tofu with rice noodles
Nutty tofu risotto
Wheat-free pizza
Red lentil dahl with rice and salad

Snack list (reduced-grain)

Rice cakes or Glutafin crackers and peanut butter or low-sugar jam
Fresh fruit, nuts and seeds
Nuts and raisins
Yogurt (live or soy)
Fruit
Dried fruit bars, such as Granovita
La Fruit – dried fruit cubes
Raw vegetables and dips, such as hoummus or taramasalata with corn
    wafers (Nachips)
Corn pasta or rice salad
Rice cakes with almond butter or pure fruit spread
Fresh fruit salad
Nuts and seeds (pecans, almonds, sunflower, sesame)
Soy yogurt (natural or fruit)
Barkat rice bread with almond butter
Cold rice salad with cottage cheese, fruit and nuts
Slice of phyto fruit loaf
Soy and linseed bread sandwich

Beverage list (reduced grains)

Hot
Redbush herbal tea
Dandelion coffee (instant or root)
Fennel tea
Ginseng tea
Raspberry and ginseng tea
Chicory drink
Other herbal teas
Lemon and ginger tea
Fennel tea
Barley cup

Cold
Mineral water
Fruit juice
Aqua Libra or Amé
Small amounts of carbonated water with fruit juice, such as Irish
    Spring, Appletise etc.
Ginger cordial

WILL YOU BE ON A RESTRICTED DIET FOR EVER?

There seems to be a definite difference between 'food allergy' and 'food sensitivity'. We often find that severe menopause cases are suffering from food sensitivity rather than actual allergy, although there are cases where women are violently allergic to certain types of food.

Realistically, if you are suffering with severe symptoms, you need to give your body a complete rest for a minimum of two to three months. We often find it takes as much as six months to a year before the body is really back to normal and can once again cope fully with foods that have been eliminated.

If you notice unpleasant side-effects occurring when you begin to reintroduce the grains, one by one, discontinue them for another month or two before attempting to reintroduce them again. Usually, the very fact that you have made so much progress is an incentive to continue with the nutritional programme.

Occasionally, we have found that some women have what seems to be a permanent allergy to a particular food which, when reintroduced, continues to make them feel very unwell. In these cases the women themselves usually decide that it's better to be well and do without the food in question than to suffer unnecessarily.

All the women who go through the programme cheat at some point. Not only do we expect it, we also think it's a positive step. It's only when you have put the system to the test yourself that you really begin to follow it because you believe in it rather than because someone else said it might work.

You begin to feel so well on the diet that you start to doubt that you really have food sensitivities. So you decide to blow the diet. You eat and enjoy one or two days' helpings of the 'forbidden fruit'. Sometimes the symptoms return within an hour or two, sometimes they creep on within a day or so; either way, you have the symptoms back again and you remember what it was like to feel so unwell. You now realise that dietary factors and your symptoms are clearly related. So it's back on the diet with a far more self-determined resolution not to cheat.

WHAT ABOUT THE LONG TERM?

Once you have followed the dietary and supplement recommendations closely for three or four months and you have noticed a substantial improvement, you can then start to relax a bit. As long as you follow the basic recommendations most of the time, the occasional indulgence should not hurt. Make sure it's only occasional to begin with and preferably not when you have a heavy schedule or pressing engagements. The dietary regime should be followed and the supplements taken until you feel your symptoms are well under control, which may take as little as three or four months or as long as nine months to a year. Once your menopause symptoms are under control, if you cannot or do not intend to take HRT, then you should continue with the supplements that are intended to help bone-regeneration. It's important to ease off the diet slowly, as a sudden withdrawal can often lead to a recurrence of the symptoms.

Occasionally, months after completing your programme, symptoms may recur. If you suspect this is happening, take some speedy action to get them under control again. Times of great stress and general illness may, in some circumstances, place extra nutritional demands on your body and this may bring on some of the old symptoms. Should this happen, return to the basic diet for a few months until things have settled down.

PART FIVE

RECIPE ROUND-UP

20
NUTRITIOUS RECIPES

It is important to think carefully about the method of cooking, as so many vital nutrients may be lost in the cooking process.

- Steam, stir-fry or grill for preference, and with as little extra fat as possible. Shallow- and deep-frying are the least healthy cooking methods as they use a lot of fat.
- Boiling is another method to be avoided if you can. With vegetables in particular, you can expect to lose over 50 per cent of the nutrients in the water.
- Vegetables are a special case: steam them over boiling water, or cook gently in a very little water.
- If you cook vegetables in boiling water from the start, you will lose fewer nutrients than if you started with cold water.
- Baking, braising and roasting are also acceptable ways of cooking. Again, use as little fat as possible.
- Braise prepared vegetables, on top of the stove or in the oven, in as little liquid as possible, only until they are *al dente*. You can add flavourings (such as garlic, onion, herbs, spices, seeds etc.) if you like.
- One way of preserving most of a food's nutrients is by using a pressure-cooker.

The recipes following include a selection of soups, salads, fish, meat and poultry, cheese and vegetables, desserts, and some breads and cakes. They should give you a fair idea of the sort of things you can still enjoy even when you are cutting down on or eliminating certain foods. All are suitable for those of you who are moderate sufferers; if you are cutting out grains, you can tell at a glance the recipes which are suitable for you. These are marked with the code WOBR, or similar. This means that the recipe is Wheat, Oat, Barley and/or Rye free.

SOUPS

Watercress Soup WOBR

SERVES 4

75 g (3 oz) watercress, washed and
  roughly chopped
3 medium sized potatoes, cubed
olive oil

550 ml (1 pint) vegetable stock
freshly ground black pepper
4 tsp fromage frais

1. Gently cook the cubes of potato in olive oil until they are soft.
2. Add the stock to the pan and simmer for 15 minutes.
3. Add the watercress and simmer for another 8 minutes. Liquidise and add the black pepper to taste.
4. Serve hot with a teaspoon of fromage frais swirled into the soup.

Cauliflower and Coriander Soup WOBR

SERVES 4

1 cauliflower
25 g (1 oz) margarine
1 onion, peeled and finely chopped
1 tsp celery seeds
1 tsp ground coriander
2 bay leaves

1 bouquet garni
900 ml (1^1/$_2$ pints) So Good soy
  milk
^{1}/$_2$ tsp Dijon mustard
freshly ground salt and black pepper

1. Chop some of the cauliflower stalk and all the florets into small pieces.
2. Melt the margarine in a large saucepan and gently sauté the onion and cubed cauliflower stalk without letting them brown.
3. Add the celery seeds, coriander, bay leaves and bouquet garni. Cook for 5 minutes, stirring occasionally.
4. Add the chopped florets and So Good, bring to the boil and simmer for 20 minutes. Remove the bay leaves and bouquet garni. Cool slightly.
5. Purée in a blender or food processor for a few seconds until creamy. Reheat in a clean saucepan. Stir in the mustard and seasoning and simmer for 2–3 minutes. Serve straight away.

Apple and Fennel Soup   WOBR

SERVES 8

500 g old potatoes, scrubbed and
  quartered
2 bulbs fennel, trimmed and
  chopped roughly
2 leeks, trimmed and chopped
2 cooking apples, cored and chopped
1 tsp sugar

1 litre (2 pints) water
550 ml (1 pint) So Good soy
  milk
25 g (2 oz) sesame seeds
1 eating apple, peeled and chopped
  into small pieces
black pepper to taste

1. Put the potatoes, fennel, leeks, cooking apples, sugar, water and So
   Good in a large pan, bring to the boil and simmer until the potatoes
   and fennel are cooked.
2. Purée the mixture in a food processor. Return to the pan, add the
   sesame seeds and chopped apple, and season to taste.

Sweet Potato and Chick Pea Soup   WOBR

SERVES 12

2 tbsp sesame seeds
2 pints (1 litre) vegetable stock
juice of 1 lime
1–2 cloves garlic, crushed
1 onion, chopped

350 g (12 oz) sweet potato, peeled
  and cut into rough chunks
425 g (15 oz) can chickpeas,
  drained and rinsed
salt and freshly ground black pepper

1. Put the sesame seeds in a large, heavy-based saucepan and heat gently, stirring constantly, for 30–60 seconds or until toasted. Be careful
   not to scorch them.
2. Stir in ¹/₂ pint (300 ml) of the stock, half of the lime juice, the garlic and onion. Cover and simmer for 5–7 minutes, then uncover and
   simmer briskly until the onions and garlic are tender, and are gently
   'frying' in their own juices.
3. Add the sweet potato pieces and stir for a few minutes. Add the
   remaining stock and simmer, partially covered, for about 15 minutes
   or until the sweet potatoes are almost tender.
4. Stir in the chick peas and remaining lime juice and season with salt
   and black pepper. Simmer, partially covered, for about 10 minutes or
   until the potatoes are tender. Cool slightly.
5. Purée the soup, in small batches, in a blender until smooth and vel-
   vety. Return to a saucepan and heat through, taste, and adjust the
   seasonings before serving.

SALADS

Watercress, Fennel and Lemon Salad WOBR

SERVES 4

1 large fennel bulb, thinly sliced
1 small bunch watercress, washed
   and trimmed
a handful of fresh parsley, washed,
   dried and finely chopped

freshly ground black pepper
1 tbsp lemon juice
$^1/_2$ lemon, thinly sliced

1. Mix together the fennel, watercress and chopped parsley.
2. Add the black pepper and the lemon juice.
3. Cut each lemon slice into segments, and add to the salad.

Carrot & Cashew Nut Coleslaw WOBR

SERVES 4

1 large carrot, grated
1 small onion, finely chopped
2 celery stalks, chopped
$^1/_4$ small, hard white cabbage,
   shredded
1 tbsp chopped fresh parsley

4 tbsp sesame oil
$^1/_2$ tsp poppy seeds
50 g (2 oz) cashew nuts
2 tbsp cider vinegar
freshly ground black pepper

1. In a large bowl, mix together the carrot, onion, celery and cabbage. Stir in the chopped parsley and season with the pepper.
2. Heat the sesame oil in a saucepan. Add the poppy seeds and cover the pan. Cook over a medium-high heat until the seeds start to make a popping sound. Remove from the heat and leave to cool.
3. Scatter the cashew nuts onto a baking tray, place them under a grill and toast until lightly browned, being careful not to burn them. Leave to cool.
4. Add the vinegar to the oil and poppy seed mixture, then pour it over the carrot mixture. Add the cooled cashew nuts. Toss together to coat with the dressing.
5. Serve with rice cakes, cold meat or oily fish.

Cottage Cheese Fruit Salad   WOBR

SERVES 4

1 lettuce, washed and shredded
4 tomatoes, cut into wedges
half a cucumber, cut into small
  cubes

2 carrots, grated
350 g (12 oz) natural cottage cheese
2 peaches, sliced and cubed
75g (3 oz) walnuts, chopped

1. Place the lettuce, tomatoes and cucumber into a large bowl.
2. Combine the cottage cheese, carrots and peaches and place on top
   of the salad.
3. Sprinkle with chopped walnuts.

Bean Salad   WOBR

SERVES 4 AS A SIDE SALAD

100 g (4 oz) podded broad beans
100 g (4 oz) canned red kidney
  beans
100 g (4 oz) haricot beans, soaked
  overnight
100 g (4 oz) chickpeas, soaked
  overnight
1 bay leaf
2 sprigs fresh thyme

1 clove garlic, peeled and crushed
  (optional)
2 tbsp cold-pressed olive or
  vegetable oil
2 tbsp finely chopped parsley
$^1/_2$ tsp cumin seeds, ground
1 medium onion, peeled and finely
  chopped

1. Cook the broad beans for 5 minutes, then drain and cool. If large,
   take off the outer skin to reveal the green inner bean. Rinse and
   drain the kidney beans.
2. Drain the haricot beans and chickpeas and cover with water in a
   saucepan. Boil for 10 minutes and then add the bay leaf and sprigs
   of thyme and simmer for $1-1^1/_2$ hours. Drain and leave to cool.
3. Mix the garlic with the oil and kidney and broad beans. Pour over
   the remaining beans.
4. Add and mix in the parsley, cumin seeds and onion.

Alfalfa and Cress Salad

WOBR

SERVES 4

2 cartons cress
100 g (4 oz) alfalfa sprouts
225 g (8 oz) cooked ham, thinly
  sliced*
4 eggs, hard-boiled, shelled and
  chopped

YOGURT DRESSING
150 ml (5 fl oz) natural yogurt
1 tbsp chopped green olives
1 tbsp chopped fresh parsley
freshly ground black pepper

1. Cut the cress from the carton and place in a mixing bowl with the alfalfa sprouts.
2. Add the ham to the salad with the chopped eggs and combine well.
3. Mix together all the dressing ingredients. Pour the dressing over the salad and toss until everything is well coated.
4. Serve the salad on its own or with crusty bread.

*the ham can be omitted for a vegetarian option

Pineapple and Watercress Salad

WOBR

SERVES 4

100 g (4 oz) watercress
1 small pineapple
50 g (2 oz) walnut halves

DRESSING
2 tbsp clear honey
2 tbsp walnut oil
2 tbsp wine vinegar
freshly ground black pepper

1. Wash the watercress and remove any coarse stalks.
2. Cut the pineapple into small cubes and combine with the watercress.
3. Mix together the dressing ingredients and pour over the salad.

Ginger and Carrot Salad

WOBR

SERVES 4 AS A SIDE SALAD

175 g (6 oz) carrots, grated
2 medium apples, grated

1 tsp ground ginger
1 celery stick, chopped

1. Toss together and serve.

Basic Dressing   WOBR

2 tbsp red or white wine   salt and freshly ground black pepper
  vinegar   4 tbsp good olive oil

1. Mix the vinegar with seasonings to taste, and then whisk in the olive oil, until the simple dressing is well emulsified.

Oil and Fruit Dressing   WOBR

MAKES 75 ML (2^1/$_2$ FL OZ)

2 tbsp olive oil   juice of 1 lemon or 1 tbsp white
1 tbsp sesame oil   wine vinegar
1 tsp mayonnaise   1 tsp concentrated apple juice
1 tsp mustard   (optional)
                                  freshly ground black pepper to taste

1. Blend all the ingredients together until smooth.
2. This dressing keeps well in the fridge in a sealed container.

Green Mayonnaise 1   WOBR

SERVES 2

1 egg, size 2   150 ml (^{1}/$_4$ pint) salad oil
1 large garlic clove, peeled and 1 spring onion, chopped, or 2 tsp
  crushed   chopped onion
^{1}/$_4$ tsp salt   75 g (3 oz) watercress, washed and
freshly ground pepper   stalks removed

1. Put the egg, garlic, salt and pepper into a liquidiser and blend together.
2. Add the oil very gradually.
3. Add the chopped onion and half the watercress. Continue to process.
4. Work in the remaining watercress. Adjust the seasoning.

Green Mayonnaise 2   WOBR

SERVES 2

1 bunch watercress, washed   lemon juice
150 ml (^{1}/$_4$ pint) very thick   salt and freshly ground pepper
  mayonnaise

1. Reserve a little watercress for garnish. Boil the remainder in a very small quantity of water. Drain and blend to a purée, then push through a sieve.
2. Add the watercress purée to the mayonnaise. Adjust the seasoning with lemon juice, salt and pepper.

FISH, POULTRY AND MEAT

Poached Salmon with Green Mayonnaise   WOBR

SERVES 2

2 salmon steaks
1 tbsp oil
salt and freshly ground pepper
lemon juice

GARNISH
Green Mayonnaise (see page 269)
lemon wedges
cucumber chunks
sprigs of watercress

1. Wipe and oil the steaks. Season with salt, pepper and lemon juice. Wrap the fish in oiled foil. Have ready a poacher, or a pan of simmering water.
2. Poach the fish for 8–10 minutes until the flesh is opaque, and a creamy curd is visible between the flakes.
3. Carefully remove the skin and bone from the fish but do not break up. Re-wrap in the foil and allow to get cold.
4. Put the salmon on a dish, and place a spoonful of green mayonnaise on each steak, or coat with the mayonnaise. Garnish with the salad ingredients.

Salmon Steaks with Ginger   WOBR

SERVES 2

2 salmon steaks
2 tbsp lemon juice
2.5 cm (1 inch) square of fresh

ginger, peeled and finely chopped
freshly ground black pepper
to taste

1. Place each salmon steak on a large piece of foil. Add 1 tablespoon lemon juice and half the chopped ginger to each steak. Season with a little black pepper.
2. Wrap the steaks individually in foil to make two parcels and bake in a preheated oven at 180°C (350°F) Gas Mark 4 for 20 minutes. Serve hot with vegetables or cold with salad.

Trout and Almonds

WOBR

SERVES 2

2 trout	25 g (1 oz) almonds, sliced
salt and freshly ground pepper	4 tbsp dry white wine
1 tbsp potato flour	GARNISH
50 g (2 oz) butter	lemon wedges
1 tbsp oil	watercress

1. Wash, clean and dry the trout, leaving the heads on.
2. Sprinkle with salt and pepper, then dip in seasoned flour.
3. Heat half the butter and the oil in a large frying pan until sizzling. Put the trout in and fry for 3 minutes on each side. Continue to cook gently on the second side until cooked. Put the fish in a dish and keep hot.
4. Heat the remaining butter in a small pan, add the almonds and fry until golden brown.
5. Pour the wine over the almonds, heat, and then pour the sauce over the trout. Garnish with lemon wedges and watercress.

Lemony Cod and Spinach Bake

OBR

SERVES 4

700 g (1 1/2 lb) cod fillets	grated rind and juice of 1 lemon
330 ml (1/2 pint) So Good soy milk	25 g (1 oz) cornflour
1 tsp tarragon	25 g (1 oz) wholemeal
freshly ground black pepper	breadcrumbs
450 g (1 lb) fresh spinach, stalks	25 g (1 oz) red Leicester cheese,
removed	grated

1. Put the cod into a saucepan and add the So Good, tarragon and pepper. Bring to the boil, reduce the heat and simmer for 10–15 minutes or until tender.
2. Place the spinach in a saucepan with 1 tablespoon of water and simmer until soft (about 10 minutes). Strain off excess liquid and season with black pepper.
3. Remove the fish from the saucepan and take off any skin. Add the lemon rind and juice to the milk. Mix the cornflour with a little cold water and stir into the So Good. Return to the heat and bring to the boil, stirring. Simmer gently for a few minutes. Flake the cod and add to the sauce.
4. Put half the spinach in the base of a large ovenproof dish and pour the fish sauce on top. Repeat the layers.
5. Mix together the breadcrumbs and cheese and sprinkle over the top

of the fish. Place under a hot grill for about 5 minutes until golden and crisp on top.

Cheesy Prawn Bake   WOBR

SERVES 4

6 hard-boiled eggs
25 g (1 oz) sunflower margarine
25 g (1 oz) cornflour
300 ml (¹/₂ pint) So Good soy milk
3 tbsp fresh parsley, chopped

freshly ground black pepper
¹/₂ tsp mustard powder
30 g (10 oz) peeled prawns
3 tbsp Cheddar or Emmenthal
  cheese, grated

1. Shell and slice the eggs.
2. Melt the margarine in a pan and stir in the cornflour. Cook, stirring for 1 minute. Remove from the heat and gradually add the So Good. Bring to the boil, stirring until thickened.
3. Stir in the pepper, mustard and parsley.
4. Arrange the prawns and eggs in an ovenproof dish. Pour over the sauce and sprinkle the top with cheese. Bake for 15–20 minutes at 180°C (350°F) Gas Mark 4, until the top is golden and bubbling.

Snow Peas with Tiger Prawns   WOBR

SERVES 4

450 g (1lb) snow peas (mangetout)
450 g (1lb) uncooked tiger prawns
375 g (13 oz) broad oriental rice
  noodles
1 tsp finely chopped root ginger

3 tbsp sesame oil
2 tbsp oyster sauce
1 tsp sugar
1 tbsp sherry or white wine
fresh coriander leaves

1. Top and tail the snow peas and wash them.
2. Clean and wash the prawns and pat them dry with kitchen paper.
3. Place the noodles in boiling water and simmer gently for 3 minutes, until slightly undercooked.
4. Place the ginger and the oil in a wok and heat. Fry the snow peas briefly in the hot oil, stirring constantly. Remove and place on a warmed dish.
5. Place the tiger prawns in the wok and cook until they become pink.
6. Drain the noodles and rinse with cold water to remove the starch.
7. Return the snow peas to the wok with the prawns, add the oyster sauce and the sugar, and simmer for another minute or two.
8. Gently pour the sherry or white wine around the circumference of

the wok, and then remove peas and prawns from the wok with a slotted spoon and transfer to a dish.

9. Place noodles in the wok and quickly stir-fry them in the remaining oil, turning constantly. Turn out onto a flat platter and place the snow peas and prawns on the top. Decorate with fresh coriander and serve immediately.

Variation
If you like spicy food, before stir-frying the noodles, mix 1 teaspoon chilli sauce with the hot oil and then place the noodles in the wok.

Prawn Provençale   WOBR

SERVES 4

675 g (1¹/₂ lb) peeled prawns
50 g (2 oz) margarine
2 tbsp olive oil
4 shallots, peeled and finely chopped
1 garlic clove, peeled and crushed
(optional)

6 tomatoes, blanched, skinned and
chopped
50 g (2 oz) tomato purée
1 tsp dried thyme
1 pinch dried basil
freshly ground black pepper

1. In a large frying pan heat the margarine with the oil. Add the shallots and garlic and fry them for 4 minutes.
2. Add the skinned tomatoes, tomato purée, thyme, basil and pepper to taste. Cover the pan, reduce the heat to low and simmer for 20 minutes.
3. Stir in the prawns and cook uncovered for a further 4 minutes. Remove from the heat and serve at once.

Tuna Jackets   WOBR

SERVES 4

1 tbsp sunflower oil
1 red, 1 yellow and 1 green pepper,
cored, seeded and diced
4 tbsp white wine vinegar
2 tbsp wholegrain mustard

1 x 200 g (7 oz) can tuna in oil,
drained and flaked
1 x 100 g (4 oz) can sweetcorn,
drained
4 hot baked potatoes
freshly ground black pepper

1. Heat the oil in a pan, add the diced pepper and sauté for 5 minutes.
2. Add the vinegar and mustard and cook for 5 minutes, stirring. Stir in the flaked tuna and sweetcorn.

3. Cut the tops off the potatoes and scoop out the centres. Chop the potato centres and stir into half the pepper relish mixture. Season with black pepper to taste.
4. Spoon the potato mixture back into the potato jackets. Serve the remaining relish separately.

Sardine Pâté   OBR

100 g (4 oz) can sardines in tomato sauce
200 g (7 oz) low-fat soft cream cheese

50 g (2 oz) fresh breadcrumbs
dash of Tabasco sauce

1. Put the sardines into a food processor with all the other ingredients.
2. Blend to a smooth paste and spoon into a serving dish. Chill in the fridge for at least 1 hour before serving.
3. Garnish with herbs, serve with oatcakes or bread and a salad.

Chicken with Almonds   WOBR

SERVES 4

4 chicken breasts
15 g (1/2 oz) butter or margarine
150 ml (1/4 pint) water

a few black peppercorns
75 g (3 oz) flaked almonds

1. Skin the chicken and brush with melted butter or margarine.
2. Place water and peppercorns in an ovenproof dish. Place the chicken in the water and cover with foil. Bake for 15 minutes in the preheated oven at 180°C (350°F) Gas Mark 4.
3. Remove the foil and sprinkle with flaked almonds. Return to the oven for a further 15 minutes, or until the chicken is tender and the almonds have browned.
4. Serve with steamed vegetables, e.g. new potatoes and broccoli.

Chicken and Leek Sauté

SERVES 4

4 chicken breasts, skinned and boned
1 tbsp sunflower oil
450 g (1 lb) leeks, finely sliced

450 ml (3/4 pint) So Good soy milk
cornflour to thicken
freshly ground black pepper

1. Heat the sunflower oil in a large frying pan and sauté the chicken

breasts until just golden. Remove from the pan and place in an ovenproof dish.
2. Sauté the leeks until soft but not browned and then add to the chicken in the dish.
3. Pour the So Good over the chicken and leeks and bake for about 45 minutes at 190°C (375°F) Gas Mark 5 until the chicken is cooked through and the leeks are tender.
4. Remove the dish from the oven and thicken the sauce with the cornflour which has been blended with a little cold water.
5. Serve the chicken, leeks and sauce with plain boiled rice and mixed fresh vegetables.

Noisettes of Lamb with Cumin and Garlic   WOBR

SERVES 3–4

1 best end of neck, boned and cut
  into 6–8 noisettes
2 tsp finely chopped fresh ginger
3–4 garlic cloves, peeled and crushed
2 tbsp ground cumin
3 tbsp olive oil

salt and freshly ground pepper
GARNISH
pomegranate seeds
brown rice, studded with raisins
chopped chives

1. Combine the ginger, garlic, cumin, oil and seasonings in a bowl and coat the lamb in this on all sides. Marinate in fridge for up to 3 hours.
2. Place the noisettes on a roasting rack and roast in the oven pre-heated to 200°C (400°F) Gas Mark 6 for 15–25 minutes depending on size, until brown on the outside but still pink in the centre.
3. Serve the noisettes with pomegranate seeds and raisin-studded rice. Garnish with chives.

Fragrant Lamb   WOBR

SERVES 6

2–3 lb (1–1.5 kg) fillet end of
  leg of lamb
3 tbsp sesame oil
1 clove garlic, chopped
1 cm (1/2 inch) piece root ginger,
  chopped
1 spring onion

1–2 tbsp light soy sauce
2 tbsp brandy
3 tbsp white wine
freshly ground black pepper
1 tsp cornflour
fresh coriander

1. Seal the lamb briefly in the hot sesame oil.

2. Remove and place in a pressure cooker with the sesame oil, garlic, ginger, spring onion, soy sauce, brandy and white wine, and season with black pepper.

3. Close the pressure cooker and bring to the boil. Lower the heat and cook for 35 minutes. Alternatively, place the ingredients plus 150 ml ($^1/_4$ pint) water in a covered dish and bake for about $1^1/_2$–2 hours at 180°C (350°F) Gas Mark 4; check liquid during cooking, adding water if needed.

4. Remove the pressure cooker from the heat and cool under running water. Place the leg of lamb on a chopping board and slice. Arrange on a serving dish, cover loosely with foil and keep warm while preparing the sauce.

5. Drain the meat juices from the pressure cooker or dish, strain into a clean pan and mix with the cornflour. Over a moderate heat thicken the sauce, stirring constantly.

6. Remove the lamb from the oven, and pour the sauce over it. Decorate with fresh coriander and serve immediately.

Spiced Lamb with Spinach
WOBR

SERVES 4

900 g (2 lb) boned leg of lamb
6 tbsp bio natural yogurt
1 cm ($^1/_2$ inch) piece of fresh root
  ginger, peeled and chopped
2 garlic cloves, crushed
2.5 cm (1 inch) cinnamon stick
2 bay leaves
2 green cardamoms

4 black peppercorns
3 whole cloves
1 tsp ground cumin
1 tsp garam masala
1 tsp chilli powder
1 tsp ground coriander
450 g (1lb) fresh spinach

1. Cut the meat into cubes, trimming off excess fat. Put the meat into a bowl and set aside. In a separate bowl, mix together the yogurt, ginger, garlic and whole and ground spices.

2. Spoon the mixture over the meat and mix thoroughly. Cover and leave to marinate at room temperature for about 4 hours.

3. Meanwhile, thoroughly wash and chop the fresh spinach.

4. Put the marinated meat in a heavy-based saucepan and cook over a low heat for about 1 hour, stirring occasionally, until all the moisture has evaporated and the meat is tender.

5. Stir in the spinach and cook over a low heat for a further 10 minutes. Serve garnished with mint and lemon slices, accompanied by boiled rice and a yogurt dressing.

Liver Pâté

WOBR

SERVES 4–6

225 g (8 oz) lambs' liver, cut into
  small pieces
slices of streaky bacon sufficient to
  line tin
50 g (2 oz) butter
1 small onion, peeled and chopped
100 g (4 oz) streaky bacon, chopped

2 level tsp cornflour
4 tbsp So Good soya milk
1 thick slice white bread or 40g
  (1½ oz) breadcrumbs
salt and freshly ground pepper
garlic salt (optional) or 1 clove
  garlic, peeled and crushed

1. Remove the rind from the bacon slices, then stretch and use to line a small bread tin or a 600 ml (1 pint) ovenproof dish.
2. Melt the butter, and fry the onion and chopped bacon gently for 5 minutes.
3. Put the onion, bacon and liver into the liquidiser.
4. Stir the flour into the remaining fat to make a roux, then slowly whisk in the SoGood to make a sauce.
5. Add this sauce and the breadcrumbs to the mixture in liquidiser, and blend for 30 seconds. Season with salt, pepper and garlic.
6. Place in the prepared bacon-lined container. Put into a bain-marie containing 2 cm (³/₄ inch) cold water. Cook in the centre of the oven preheated to 180°C (350°F) Gas Mark 4 for 40 minutes. Leave in the tin to cool.
7. Turn out when cold. Garnish with salad ingredients, olives or gherkins and serve with slices of hot toast.

CHEESE AND VEGETABLES

Spinach and Egg Gratin

OBR

SERVES 4

900 g (2 lb) spinach
3 hard-boiled eggs, sliced
50 g (2 oz) margarine
50 g (2 oz) cornflour

450 ml (³/₄ pint) So Good soy milk
freshly ground black pepper
2 tbsp fresh brown breadcrumbs
50 g (2 oz) Cheddar cheese, grated

1. Cook the spinach in boiling water until just wilted, and drain. Put half the spinach in a greased ovenproof dish, place the eggs on top and cover with the remaining spinach.
2. Melt the margarine in a pan, stir in the flour and cook gently,

stirring. Remove from the heat and gradually add the So Good, stirring continuously. Return to the heat and bring to the boil. Cook, stirring until thickened. Season to taste.

3. Pour the sauce over the spinach and sprinkle with the breadcrumbs and cheese. Bake at 220°C (425°F) Gas Mark 7 for 15 minutes until golden brown. Serve with potatoes and fresh vegetables.

Chickpea Dips   WOBR

SERVES 8

2 x 425 g (15 oz) cans chickpeas,
  drained and rinsed
1 garlic clove, peeled and crushed
1 tbsp fresh lemon juice
25 ml (1 fl oz) olive oil
175 ml (6 fl oz) Greek plain yogurt
freshly ground black pepper
4 tsp freshly chopped parsley

2 tsp tomato purée
TO GARNISH AND SERVE
sprigs of parsley
strips of red pepper
pieces of sliced lemon
a selection of raw vegetables
  (peppers, radishes, carrots, celery
  and cucumber)

1. Place the chickpeas in a blender or food processor and blend until smooth.
2. Add the garlic, lemon juice, olive oil and yogurt and mix well. Add black pepper to taste.
3. Transfer one-third of the mixture to a small serving bowl – this will remain plain. Divide the rest between another 2 small mixing bowls.
4. Add the chopped parsley to one of these, stir well and transfer to a small serving bowl.
5. Add the tomato purée to the other, stir well and transfer to a small serving bowl. Adjust the seasoning if necessary.
6. Garnish the herb dip with sprigs of parsley, the tomato dip with red pepper and the plain dip with pieces of lemon.
7. Chop the raw vegetables into sticks. Arrange on a serving dish around the dips.

Stir-fry Vegetables   WOBR

There are many different vegetable in season that can be used for stir-frying. You can use six or seven different vegetables, or only two or three. To obtain the best results, stir-fry vegetables should be cooked with the minimum oil at a high heat, to seal in the flavour.

There are many nice last-minute additions to your stir-fry. Experiment to find your favourite seasoning and flavouring. Less well-known ingredients are available from health-food shops.

Seasonings
Salt, pepper, chilli, grated ginger, five-spice powder (use very moderately), sesame seeds (ground), fenugreek (ground), turmeric, coriander, paprika, nori seaweed (toasted and crumbled).

Flavourings
Shoyu/tamari (wheat-free alternative to soy sauce), miso, sesame oil, tahini (sesame seed paste), sherry, vermouth, lemon juice.

SERVES 4 WITH NOODLES OR RICE   WOBR

450 g (1lb) fresh broccoli
225 g (8 oz) cauliflower
1 tbsp oil
2.5 cm (1 inch) fresh root ginger,
  sliced and finely shredded
2 large carrots, peeled and sliced
$^1/_2$ tsp sesame oil
225 g (8 oz) fresh beansprouts
225 g (8 oz) Chinese leaves or
  white cabbage, shredded
$^1/_2$ tsp salt

1. Separate the broccoli heads into small florets and peel and slice the stems. Separate the cauliflower florets and slice stems.
2. Heat the oil in a large wok or frying pan. When it is moderately hot add ginger shreds. Stir-fry for a few seconds.
3. Add the carrots, cauliflower and broccoli and stir-fry for 2–3 minutes, then add the sesame oil, beansprouts and Chinese leaves or white cabbage. Stir-fry for further 2–3 minutes.
4. Season to taste, and serve at once.

Garlic can be substituted for ginger, and tamari sauce can be added in the final stage of frying before serving.

Broccoli with Coconut and Cashews WOBR

SERVES 4

200 g (7 oz) creamed coconut
300 ml (¹/₂ pint) boiling water
275 g (10 oz) broccoli, stalks sliced
  and tops broken into florets
1 tbsp sunflower oil
1 medium onion, finely chopped

2.5 cm (1 inch) piece of fresh root
  ginger, peeled and finely chopped
75 g (3 oz) cashew nuts
1 tsp ground turmeric
2 tsp ground coriander
freshly ground black pepper to taste

1. Put the coconut in a bowl, pour over the boiling water and stir until dissolved.
2. Steam or parboil the broccoli for 2–3 minutes, then rinse under cold running water and drain.
3. Heat the oil in a wok or frying pan until hot. Add the onion, ginger, cashews, turmeric and coriander and stir-fry gently for 2–3 minutes, without browning.
4. Add the coconut milk and pepper to taste, then simmer gently for 2–3 minutes or until the mixture thickens.
5. Add the broccoli and simmer for a further 2 minutes. Serve immediately with rice or noodles.

Brown Lentil Scotch Eggs WOBR

SERVES 4

1 ¹/₂ tbsp sunflower oil
2 large onions, peeled and finely
  chopped
1 garlic clove, peeled and crushed
175 g (6 oz) brown lentils, cooked
  and drained well
1 tbsp dried oregano

1 tbsp basil
1 tbsp lemon juice
freshly ground black pepper to taste
1 egg, beaten
4 small eggs, hard-boiled and shelled
1 tbsp sesame seeds

1. Heat half the oil in a frying pan and gently fry the onions for 6–8 minutes.
2. Add the garlic, lentils, oregano, basil, lemon juice and black pepper, and mix well with a fork until the mixture binds together. If necessary, add some of the beaten egg.
3. Dip each boiled egg into the beaten egg mixture and cover with one quarter of the lentil mixture. Brush again with beaten egg and roll in seeds. Repeat this procedure with each egg.
4. Cut 4 squares of foil, large enough to wrap each egg in. Brush each

of these squares with the remaining oil, then wrap around the eggs. Place on a baking tray and bake in the preheated oven at 180°C (350°F) Gas Mark 4 for 15 minutes.

5. Remove the foil carefully and serve the eggs hot or cold.

Nutty Tofu Risotto   WOBR

SERVES 4

225 g (8 oz) brown rice
1 tbsp sunflower oil
1 medium onion, peeled and chopped
1 garlic clove, peeled and crushed
1 red pepper, seeded and sliced
1 green pepper, seeded and sliced
50 g (2 oz) green beans
100 g (4 oz) carrots, cut into matchsticks

100 g (4 oz) courgettes, thinly sliced
100 g (4 oz) broccoli, broken into florets and stalk sliced
225 g (8 oz) tofu, chopped
1 small seedless orange, peeled and segmented
1 tbsp flaked almonds
1 tbsp fresh chopped parsley

1. Cook the rice as directed on the packet and put to one side.
2. Heat the oil in a large frying pan and add the onion, garlic, red and green peppers and fry gently for 2–3 minutes.
3. Steam the beans, carrots, courgettes, and broccoli over a pan of boiling water for 5 minutes (alternatively miss the steaming if you like your vegetables crunchy). Add to the other ingredients in the frying pan.
4. Add the tofu, orange segments, flaked almonds, parsley and rice and heat through until all the ingredients are hot. Serve immediately.

Bean and Tomato Hotpot   WOBR

SERVES 4

2 tbsp sunflower oil
2 onions, peeled and sliced
3 carrots, sliced
2 celery sticks, sliced
1 large leek, sliced
2 garlic cloves, peeled and crushed
1 x 425 g (15 oz) can red kidney beans, drained

1 x 400 g (14 oz) can chopped tomatoes
300 ml (1/2 pint) vegetable stock
1 tbsp yeast extract
freshly ground black pepper
675 g (1 1/2 lb) potatoes, peeled and thinly sliced
15 g (1/2 oz) margarine

1. Heat the oil in a flameproof casserole, add the onions and fry for 5 minutes. Add the carrots, celery, leek and garlic and fry for a further 5 minutes.

2. Add the kidney beans, tomatoes with their juices, stock, yeast extract and pepper to taste. Mix well.

3. Arrange the potatoes neatly on top, sprinkling pepper between each layer. Dot with the margarine, cover and cook in the oven preheated to 180°C (350°F) Gas Mark 4 for 2 hours.

4. Remove the lid 30 minutes before the end of cooking to allow the potatoes to brown.

Oat and Almond Bake

BR

SERVES 6

50 g (2 oz) porridge oats
50 g (2 oz) whole green lentils
225 g (8 oz) leeks
225 g (8 oz) carrots
100 g (4 oz) celery
1 parsnip
1 green pepper
1 tbsp oil
1 tsp thyme
1/2 tsp mustard powder

SAUCE
50 g (2 oz) ground almonds
150 ml (1/4 pint) water
150 ml (1/4 pint) So Good soy milk
25 g (1 oz) cornflour
freshly ground black pepper
TOPPING
50 g (2 oz) porridge oats
50 g (2 oz) fresh breadcrumbs
1 tbsp sunflower seeds

1. Wash the lentils then place them in a large pan of water (approx 1 litre/2 pints), and boil for 45 minutes. Drain the lentils 3 times to ensure that the starch is removed.

2. Chop the vegetables finely, then sauté them in the oil so they are coated. Pour in about a cup of water and cook for 10–15 minutes until the vegetables are just tender, but not soft.

3. Mix in the thyme, mustard and well-drained lentils. Cook for another 5 minutes.

4. Meanwhile make the sauce. Mix the ground almonds with the remaining water and So Good. Melt the margarine in a pan, stir in the cornflour and cook for 1 minute.

5. Pour in the almond milk mixture, stirring continuously. Bring to the boil and season to taste.

6. Pour the sauce over the cooked vegetables, then turn into an oven-proof dish.

7. Mix the topping ingredients together and sprinkle over the top.

8. Bake at 180°C (350°F) Gas Mark 4 for 20 minutes, until browned on top. Serve with extra fresh vegetables.

Vegetable Lasagne   OBR

SERVES 6

1 carrot, peeled and chopped
1 large onion, peeled and sliced
1 red pepper, seeded and chopped
1 green pepper, seeded and chopped
1 large aubergine, cut into chunks
225 g (8 oz) button mushrooms,
   sliced
1 large courgette, sliced
2 tbsp olive oil
1 garlic clove, peeled and crushed
1 tbsp paprika

2 tsp dried marjoram
2 x 400 g (14 oz) cans chopped
   tomatoes
2 tbsp tomato purée
2 bay leaves
freshly ground black pepper
350 g (12 oz) fresh lasagne
900 ml (1½ pints) béchamel sauce
   (see page 288)
3 tbsp freshly grated Parmesan or
   Cheddar cheese (optional)

1. Heat the oil in a saucepan. Add the garlic, carrot, onion and peppers and fry for 1–2 minutes. Add paprika, marjoram and aubergine. Fry for 1–2 minutes.
2. Add the mushrooms and courgette to the pan with the tomatoes and juices, tomato purée, bay leaves and black pepper. Bring to the boil, reduce the heat, cover and simmer for 30 minutes.
3. Spread a small amount of the tomato sauce in the base of a 3 litre (5 pint) ovenproof dish. Cover with a layer of lasagne and top with a layer of béchamel sauce. Repeat these layers once more, finishing off with a layer of béchamel sauce.
4. Sprinkle with the cheese if using. Bake in the preheated oven at 190°C (375°F) Gas Mark 5 for 45–50 minutes until well browned.

Watercress Mousse   WOBR

SERVES 4

2 bunches watercress
7 g (¼ oz) vegetarian gelatine powder
4 tbsp hot chicken stock
100 g (4 oz) Philadelphia cream
   cheese

4 tbsp mayonnaise
salt and freshly ground pepper
a dash of Tabasco sauce (or
   cayenne pepper)
4 tbsp double cream

1. Dissolve the gelatine in the hot stock, then leave to cool.
2. Remove and discard half the stalks from the watercress, then wash and dry the remainder of the leaves and stalks.
3. Purée all but 4 sprigs of the watercress with the dissolved gelatine. Add the cheese, mayonnaise and seasoning. Blend thoroughly.
4. Whip the cream until it holds soft peaks, then fold into the purée.

5. Pour into four small dishes, and allow to set.
6. Just before serving, garnish with the reserved sprigs of watercress.

Spinach Lasagne   WOBR

SERVES 6

350 g (12 oz) fresh spinach, washed
1 tsp olive oil
1 tsp grated nutmeg
1 small red onion, diced
100 g (4 oz) mushrooms, sliced
1 clove garlic, crushed
1 tsp tamari sauce
250 g (8 oz) Ricotta cheese
25 g (1 oz) Parmesan cheese, grated
250 g (8 oz) Mascarpone cheese

100 g (4 oz) Cheddar cheese,
  grated
freshly ground black pepper
TOMATO SAUCE
1 medium onion, diced
2 tbsp olive oil
500 g (1lb) can chopped tomatoes
1 clove garlic
1 large bunch basil
freshly ground black pepper

1. Place the spinach and a little salt and pepper in a pan and cook over a low heat for 1 minute until wilted. Drain thoroughly and add a little grated nutmeg. Chop roughly and set aside to cool.
2. Heat the olive oil and, when it is very hot, add the first onion and sauté for 5–6 minutes, then add the mushrooms, garlic and tamari. Sauté for 1–2 minutes until browned. Mix with the spinach and set aside to cool. Finally mix with the Ricotta and Parmesan.
3. Make the tomato sauce: heat the oil, add the onion and sauté until transparent. Add the tinned tomatoes and garlic. Add the basil, seasoning and cook gently for about 25 minutes until all the water has evaporated and the sauce is thick. Remove the cooked basil and replace with some freshly chopped leaves.
4. Layer the sheets of lasagne in an ovenproof dish with the spinach and tomato sauce mixture, finishing with a layer of tomato sauce until all the pasta has been used.
5. Cover the top with the Mascarpone and grated Cheddar cheese and bake at 200°C (400°F) Gas Mark 6 for 25–30 minutes until the top is golden brown.

Spinach and Potato Curry

WOBR

SERVES 4

2 tbsp sunflower oil
225 g (8 oz) potatoes, peeled and
  cut into chunks
1 clove garlic, crushed
1 tsp freshly grated root ginger

1 green chilli, halved and seeded
450 g (1lb) fresh spinach, roughly
  chopped
2–3 sprigs fresh coriander leaves
pinch of freshly ground rock salt

1. Heat the oil in a pan and sauté the potatoes for 4–5 minutes. Add the garlic and ginger and chilli halves. Sauté for a further 1–2 minutes.
2. Stir in the spinach, coriander and salt. Add a little water and continue sautéing for 10–15 minutes until the potatoes are tender and the spinach is dry. Serve with basmati rice and poppadoms.

Nut and Vegetable Loaf

WOBR

SERVES 4–6

2 tsp sunflower oil
1 small onion, peeled and chopped
1 small carrot, chopped
1 celery stick, chopped
1 tbsp tomato purée
225 g (8 oz) tomatoes, skinned and
  chopped
2 eggs
1 tbsp chopped parsley
freshly ground black pepper
225 g (8 oz) shelled nuts (almonds,
  walnuts, hazelnuts, pecans),
  finely chopped or minced

GARNISH
onion rings
parsley sprigs

1. Heat the oil in a pan, and cook the onion, carrot and celery until softened. Add the tomato purée and tomatoes and cook for 5 minutes.
2. Put the eggs, parsley and pepper to taste in a bowl and beat well. Stir in the nuts and vegetables.
3. Transfer to a greased 900 ml (1¹/₂ pint) ovenproof dish and bake in the oven preheated to 220°C (425°F) Gas Mark 7 for 30–35 minutes.
4. Turn out and decorate with onion rings and parsley. Serve hot with vegetables or cold with a salad and mustard sauce (see page 288).

Tofu Loaf

SERVES 4

450 g (1 lb) tofu
3 carrots, peeled and grated
2 parsnips, peeled and grated
1 cup frozen green peas, thawed

$^1/_3$ cup ground almonds
125 g ($^1/_4$ lb) cream cheese with
  chives, softened
1 cup parsley, chopped

1. Preheat the oven to 180°C (350°F) Gas Mark 4. Combine all the ingredients except the parsley in a large bowl and mix well until thoroughly combined.
2. Put the mixture into a greased loaf tin and bake for 45–50 minutes until firm and the top is golden. Sprinkle with the remaining parsley and serve.

Cajun Tofu

SERVES 4

450 g (1 lb) firm tofu, cut into
  2.5-cm (1-inch) slices
1 clove garlic, cut in half
1 tsp paprika

1 tsp rock salt
1 tsp fresh sage
$^1/_2$ tsp cayenne pepper
$^1/_2$ tsp freshly ground black pepper

1. Rub both sides of the tofu with garlic. Combine the next 5 ingredients in a bowl.
2. Press seasoning mixture into the tofu with your hands so it is firmly adhered.
3. Heat some soy oil in a large frying pan and when it becomes piping hot, add the tofu. Reduce the heat to medium and cook 4–5 minutes either side, until the tofu is golden and cooked throughout.
4. Serve with brown rice and salad.

Wheat and Gluten-free Pizza

SERVES 4

DOUGH BASE
200 g (7 oz) Doves Farm gluten-
  free flour mix
50 g (2 oz) ground almonds
1 sachet instant dried yeast

1 tsp sugar
1 tsp salt
1 tbsp olive oil
250 ml ($^1/_2$ pint) warm water

TOPPING
4 tbsp tomato sauce (homemade or
    a jar of pasta sauce)
1 tbsp fresh or dried mixed herbs
75 g (3 oz) mushrooms, cleaned
    and thinly sliced
100 g (4 oz) courgettes, thinly sliced

50 g (2 oz) red pepper, thinly sliced
50 g (2 oz) green pepper, thinly
    sliced
2 ripe tomatoes, thinly sliced
50 g (2 oz) Mozzarella cheese
50 g (2 oz) Cheddar cheese
50 g (2 oz) Emmental cheese

1. Mix the flour with the other dough ingredients until well combined. Leave to prove for about 25 minutes in a warm place.
2. Give the mixture another stir and transfer it onto a large piece of baking parchment (this will prevent it sticking!). Spread the mixture out evenly with the back of a spoon until it is the size of a large dinner plate. The mixture is quite sticky – you cannot roll it out like normal bread dough, but don't panic!
3. Lightly sauté the mushrooms, courgettes and peppers in a little olive oil until slightly softened.
4. Spread the tomato sauce over the dough base and then sprinkle with the herbs.
5. Grate the cheese and combine in a bowl and sprinkle half over the tomato base.
6. Arrange the sautéed vegetables over the cheese and tomato mixture, then put the sliced tomatoes on top. Cover with the remaining cheese.
7. Bake for approximately 30 minutes at 180°C (350°F) Gas Mark 4 until the pizza is cooked and the topping is golden brown.
8. Serve with a large mixed salad.

You can use this recipe as a good 'base', and then add extra ingredients to give variety.

Suggested Extra Toppings
Tuna and prawns
Ham and pineapple
Salami
Chicken
Olives
Spinach

Mustard Sauce

WOBR

SERVES 4–6

If you use only the margarine, cornflour (or ordinary flour if you are not avoiding grains) milk and seasonings, you will have a béchamel sauce to use in the lasagne on page 283.

1 tbsp margarine
1 garlic clove, peeled and crushed
1 1/2 tbsp cornflour
freshly ground black pepper to taste

300 ml (1/2 pint) So Good soy milk
1 tbsp prepared French or German mustard
1 tbsp lemon juice

1. Melt the margarine in a saucepan over a moderate heat. Add the garlic and cook for 4 minutes.
2. Remove the pan from the heat and stir in the cornflour with a wooden spoon. Add the pepper and make into a smooth paste. Gradually stir in the milk, beating well to avoid lumps.
3. Stir in the mustard thoroughly.
4. Return the sauce to a low heat and cook for 3–4 minutes until it has thickened. Do not let the sauce boil.
5. Remove the pan from the heat and stir in the lemon juice. Pour into a sauce boat and serve immediately.

Tofu, Bean and Herb Stir-fry

WOBR

SERVES 4

2 tbsp vegetable oil
275 g (10 oz) tofu (bean curd) drained, dried and cut into cubes
2 garlic cloves, peeled and crushed
350 g (12 oz) green beans

3 tbsp chopped fresh herbs (thyme, parsley, chervil and chives)
4 spring onions, thinly sliced
2 tbsp soy sauce

1. Heat 1 tablespoon of oil in a wok or frying pan. When hot, add the tofu and garlic and stir-fry for 2 minutes. Lift out with a slotted spoon and drain.
2. Heat the remaining oil in the pan and when hot add the green beans and stir-fry gently for 4–5 minutes.
3. Add the herbs, spring onions and soy sauce, and stir-fry for a further minute.
4. Return the tofu to the pan and heat through for 1 minute, then serve immediately.

Herb Tofu   WOBR

SERVES 2

1 dsp vegetable oil

1 small red pepper, seeded and
thinly sliced

1 garlic clove, peeled and crushed

175 g (6 oz) tofu, cubed

$^1/_2$ tbsp chopped parsley

1. Heat the oil in a frying pan. Add the red pepper and garlic, and fry for 2–3 minutes.
2. Add the tofu and parsley and continue to stir-fry until the tofu is heated through. Serve immediately.

Red Lentil and Coconut Smoothy   WOBR

SERVES 4

225 g (8 oz) red split lentils

100 g (4 oz) carrots, sliced

1 medium onion, peeled and finely
chopped

1 garlic clove, peeled and crushed

1 tsp paprika

$^1/_2$ tsp ground ginger

1 bay leaf

$^1/_2$ oz (15 g) creamed coconut,
finely chopped

2 tbsp lemon juice

freshly ground black pepper to taste

1. Wash the lentils and put in a large saucepan with the carrot, onion, garlic, paprika, ginger, bay leaf and 600 ml (1 pint) water. Bring to the boil and remove any scum. Cover the pan and simmer for 25–30 minutes until the water has been absorbed.
2. Remove the bay leaf and mash the mixture into a smooth paste with a fork. Add the coconut, lemon juice and black pepper.
3. Serve hot with vegetables and rice.

DESSERTS

Pancakes with Lemon and Sugar   WOBR

SERVES 4

100 g (4 oz) wholemeal (or
buckwheat if avoiding wheat) flour

1 egg, medium

300 ml ($^1/_2$ pint) So Good soy milk

sunflower oil

TO SERVE

caster sugar

lemon juice

1. Make a thin batter with the flour, egg and milk.
2. Grease a small frying pan lightly with oil, and put in 2 tablespoons of batter at a time. Swirl the pan around so the batter covers the entire bottom of the pan.
3. Cook until golden, then flip over with a spatula, and cook the other side for a few seconds.
4. Keep warm in a folded teatowel while you make the remaining 7 pancakes.
5. Sprinkle each pancake with sugar and lemon juice and roll up.

Alternative fillings
Put 1 teaspoon pure fruit jam or 1 tablespoon stewed fruit or dried fruit conserve (see page 295), in the centre of each pancake, and roll up.

Soy and Rice Pancakes

WOBR

SERVES 4

50 g (2 oz) soy flour
50 g (2 oz) rice flour
300 ml (¹/₂ pint) So Good soy milk

1 egg
vegetable oil

1. Blend the flours, milk and egg in the liquidiser.
2. Grease a griddle or frying pan with a little oil and fry pancakes as described in the recipe above.

Pancakes with Raspberries and Cinnamon Cream

WOBR

SERVES 4

50 g (2 oz) cornflour
50 g (2 oz) rice flour
a pinch of salt
25 g (1 oz) caster sugar
2 eggs and 2 extra yolks
150 ml (¹/₄ pint) So Good soy milk
150 ml (¹/₄ pint) single cream
2 tbsp brandy
2 tbsp melted butter

a little vegetable oil and/or more
* melted butter*
FILLING
450 g (1 lb) raspberries,
* loganberries, blackberries,*
* strawberries or similar berry fruits*
300 ml (¹/₂ pint) double cream
2 tsp ground cinnamon sieved with
* 2 tsp icing sugar*

1. To prepare the pancake batter, sieve the flours and salt into a bowl, then stir in the sugar. Make a well in the centre, place the eggs and egg yolks in the well and gradually mix all the ingredients together.

Add the So Good and cream slowly, beating well, until a smooth batter is formed. Stir in enough brandy to make a thin cream. Leave to stand for 30 minutes.

2. Cook the raspberries for the filling, reserving a few of the best for decoration, with a little water and sugar until their juices run. Push through a sieve and sweeten to taste.

3. Whip the cream until it is thick. Sweeten and flavour with the mixed cinnamon and sugar.

4. Stir the melted butter into the batter. Lightly grease a small pancake pan with either butter or a mixture of butter and oil and fry as many thin pancakes as possible. Keep the stack of pancakes warm, covered in foil.

5. Spread each pancake with 2 tablespoons of whipped cream followed by 2 tablespoons of raspberry purée. Cover with another pancake and continue layering in the same way, ending with a pancake.

6. Decorate with the reserved raspberries and serve cut into wedges.

Rhubarb and Oat Crumble   WBR

SERVES 4–6

900 g (2 lb) fresh rhubarb	25 g (1 oz) sunflower seeds
100 g (4 oz) brown sugar	25 g (1 oz) mixed chopped nuts
50 g (2 oz) butter	1 tsp mixed spice
100 g (4 oz) rolled oats	1 tsp ground cinnamon

1. Peel and chop the rhubarb, and cook in a saucepan with 75 g (3 oz) of the sugar until tender. Place in a suitable ovenproof dish.

2. Rub together the butter and oats, then mix in the remaining sugar, sunflower seeds and mixed nuts. Sprinkle over the rhubarb.

3. Bake in the preheated oven at 180°C (350°F) Gas Mark 4 for 20 minutes, or until golden brown on the top. Serve hot, with fresh cream or yogurt.

Cinnamon Rhubarb   WOBR

SERVES 2

300 g (11 oz) rhubarb	40–50 g (1 1/2–2 oz) granulated or
4 tbsp water	muscavado sugar
a pinch of ground cinnamon	

1. Peel and chop the rhubarb, and put in a saucepan with the water, cinnamon and sugar, and stew until the rhubarb is tender.

2. Spoon into dishes and serve.

Fruit Compote
WOBR

SERVES 6

175 g (6 oz) dried apricots
100 g (4 oz) dried prunes
100 g (4 oz) dried figs
100 g (4 oz) dried apples

600 ml (1 pint) apple juice
$^1/_2$ tsp mixed spice
25 g (1 oz) coarsely chopped
   walnuts

1. Place the dried fruits in a bowl with apple juice and mixed spice and leave to soak overnight.
2. Transfer to a saucepan and simmer for 15 minutes. Divide between 4 separate dishes and sprinkle with walnuts.
3. Serve hot or cold with cream or yogurt.

Fresh Fruit Salad
WOBR

SERVES 4

1 dessert apple, peeled, cored and
   sliced
1 banana, peeled and sliced
4 tbsp lemon juice
1 orange, peeled and segmented

1 grapefruit, peeled and segmented
100 g (4 oz) seedless grapes
2 kiwi fruits, peeled and sliced
2 tbsp orange juice
4 sprigs fresh mint

1. Toss the apple and banana in the lemon juice. This will prevent discoloration.
2. Combine all the fruits in a serving bowl. Serve chilled and decorated with the sprigs of mint.

Baked custard

SERVES 4

3 eggs and 1 egg yolk
1 heaped tbsp honey

375 ml ($^3/_4$ pint) So Good soy milk
grated nutmeg (optional)

1. Lightly beat the eggs and egg yolk with the honey.
2. Pour the milk into this mixture.
3. Strain into an ovenproof dish and grate the fresh nutmeg over.
4. Stand the dish in a small roasting tin. Pour in enough water to come half-way up the sides of the dish.
5. Cook at 325°F (160°C) Gas Mark 3 for 1 hour until firm. To test, slip a knife in, and if it comes out clean, the custard is cooked.
6. Serve hot or cold with fresh fruit and cream!

Burgen Bread and Butter Pudding

SERVES 4

8 slices of Burgen bread, lightly
  buttered
50 g (2 oz) sultanas
25 g (1 oz) Linusit golden linseeds
1 tsp ground cinnamon

1 tsp ground ginger
2 tbsp demerara sugar
1 large egg
250 ml (^{1}/$_2$ pint) So Good soy milk

1. Line a deep ovenproof dish with half the bread, buttered side down
   (cut each slice of bread into 4 diagonally).
2. Sprinkle on the fruit, linseeds and half the sugar. Cover with the
   remaining bread, buttered side up.
3. Beat the egg and So Good and add the cinnamon and ginger. Pour
   this mixture over the bread and leave to stand for 30 minutes to
   soak.
4. Sprinkle with the remaining sugar and bake at 190°C (350°F) Gas
   Mark 4 for about 1 hour, or until golden.

Banana and Tofu Cream   WOBR

SERVES 4

200 g (7 oz) firm tofu
200 g (7 oz) bananas, peeled and
  sliced

75 g (3 oz) ground almonds
a pinch of ground cinnamon
2 tsp almond flakes

1. Blend or process the tofu and bananas together. To obtain a creamy
   texture the mixture may need to be put through a sieve or food mill.
2. Add the ground almonds and mix well.
3. Spoon into 4 bowls or glasses, and sprinkle lightly with cinnamon
   and a few almond flakes.

Baked Bananas   WOBR

SERVES 6

6 large bananas   1 tbsp vegetable oil

1. Preheat the oven to 160°C (325°F) Gas Mark 3.
2. Rub the banana skins with a little of the oil. Brush an ovenproof
   dish with the remaining oil.
3. Lay the bananas in the oiled dish and bake in the centre of the

preheated oven for 30–40 minutes or until the bananas are soft and the skins have turned black.

4. Serve the bananas hot, with one strip of the skin peeled back.

Almond and Raisin Cheesecake Bake

75 g (3 oz) raisins
5 tbsp natural cottage cheese
4.5 fl oz (140 ml) So Good
  soy milk
3 eggs

75 g (3 oz) unrefined sugar
zest and juice of 1 lemon
50 g (2 oz) butter
50 g (2 oz) ground almonds
icing sugar

1. Grease and line an ovenproof dish or a 1 kg (2 lb) loaf tin.
2. Sprinkle the raisins over the bottom and set aside.
3. Mix the remaining ingredients (except the icing sugar) together in a food blender until smooth.
4. Pour this mixture over the raisins and bake in a preheated oven at 190°C (375°F) Gas Mark 5 for 40–45 minutes or longer until set and firm to touch.
5. Sprinkle the top with icing sugar.

This makes a lovely dessert, served warm with natural yogurt or cream or cold, sliced as a cake.

Alternative
Replace the raisins with any soft fruit, such as mixed berries, mashed banana or puréed mango.

Rice and Almond Brûlée

550 ml (1 pint) So Good soy milk
50 g (2 oz) pudding rice
50 g (2 oz) ground almonds

3 tbsp sugar
1 tsp ground ginger
1 tsp ground cinnamon

1. Grease an ovenproof dish and pour in the So Good. Add the rice, almonds, 2 tbsp of the sugar, the cinnamon and ginger and bake at 160°C (325°F) Gas Mark 3 for 2 hours.
2. Leave the rice to cool, then sprinkle the remaining sugar over the surface.
3. Caramelise the top by placing the bowl under the grill until the sugar melts and turns a golden colour.
4. Chill well before serving, then serve warm with fruit and cream.

Apple Purée

4 medium Bramley cooking apples
water (or cider)
rind and juice of ¹/₂ lemon

50–75 g (2–3 oz) caster sugar
a pinch of ground cinnamon or
   ground ginger if liked

1. Preheat the oven to 190°C (375°F) Gas Mark 5.
2. Wipe and core the apples, then cut just through the skin around the 'equator' of each apple.
3. Place in a suitable dish and bake in the preheated oven for 35–40 minutes. Leave to cool.
4. Remove the apple pulp from the skin, and beat smooth with the other ingredients.

Apricot Purée

175 g (6 oz) dried apricots, soaked,
   stewed and drained, or 450 g (1lb)
   fresh stewed or canned apricots

juice of ¹/₂ lemon
75–100 g (3–4 oz) caster sugar

Rub the drained apricots through a nylon sieve. Add the remaining ingredients.

Dried Fruit Conserve   WOBR

SERVES 2

200 g (7 oz) dried apricots
apple juice
FLAVOURINGS
1 tsp orange-flower water

or
1 tsp grated orange peel
or
50 g (2 oz) flaked almonds

1. Soak the apricots overnight in apple juice.
2. Put the apricots into a saucepan and just cover them with apple juice, using the minimum amount to ensure a thick purée. Simmer them, uncovered, for about 30 minutes or until they are thoroughly cooked and soft.
3. Cool and thoroughly blend or sieve them until they have a smooth, thick consistency.
4. Add one of the flavourings.
5. The purée will keep in the refrigerator for about 10 days.

Caramel Custard

WOBR

SERVES 4

CARAMEL
100 g (4 oz) granulated sugar
6 tbsp water
1 tbsp hot water

CUSTARD
4 eggs
1 tbsp caster sugar
450 ml (³/4 pint) So Good soy milk
2–3 drops vanilla essence

1. Put the sugar and water for the caramel into a small saucepan. Dissolve the sugar over a gentle heat, stirring occasionally. Do not boil.
2. Wrap a folded tea-towel round a 600 ml (1 pint) soufflé dish to protect the hands.
3. When all the sugar has dissolved, boil the syrup until it turns a rich brown. At once add the hot water and pour it into the dish. Turn the dish round slowly to coat the base and sides with caramel. Leave to become cold.
4. Beat the eggs and sugar together. Warm the So Good until it steams and stir it into the beaten egg, add the vanilla. Strain the custard into the soufflé dish.
5. Cover with a piece of greased greaseproof paper and put into a roasting tin half-filled with water. Bake in the preheated oven at 160°C (325°F) Gas Mark 3 for about 1 hour. Test for set with a knife. When set, remove from the oven, and allow to become cold.
6. To turn out, loosen the top edge all around with a finger, then tilt the bowl to let the custard draw away from the sides. Invert the serving dish over the custard then turn out onto the dish. Lift the soufflé dish off carefully.

Phyto-Rich Muesli

SERVES 10–12

2 ¹/2 mugs puffed rice
2 mugs cornflakes
¹/2 mug chopped almonds
¹/2 mug pumpkin seeds
¹/2 mug chopped pecan nuts

¹/2 mug sesame seeds
¹/2 mug pine kernels
¹/3 mug organic linseeds
²/3 mug organic raisins
¹/2 mug organic apricots, chopped

I usually recommend making a large quantity of this, and storing it in a sealed container.

1. Mix the ingredients together and store in a sealed container. Serve with chopped fresh fruit and soy yogurt or So Good soy milk.

Note If you are constipated you will need to sprinkle an additional 1–2 tablespoons of organic linseeds onto your muesli each morning for the best results!

Phyto Fruit Loaf

150 g (5 oz) soya flour
100–125 g (4 oz) buckwheat flour
100–125 g (4 oz)organic linseeds
  (whole)
100–125 g (4 oz) ground almonds
50 g (2 oz) sesame seeds
50 g (2 oz) sunflower seeds
275 g (10 oz) dried fruit of your
  choice, e.g., organic raisins and
  sultanas
2 level tbsp unrefined caster sugar

1 tsp each of nutmeg and ginger
1 tbsp ground cinnamon
12 drops of ginger herb or spice
  extract (in vegetable oil)* or 2,
  2.5-cm (1-inch) squares (approx)
  stem ginger (chopped very finely)
2 heaped tsp wheat-free baking
  powder
825 ml (1^1/$_2$ pints approx) So Good
  soy milk

1. Mix all dry ingredients in a large bowl.
2. Pour the So Good over the dry ingredients and stir well.
3. Leave to stand for 1 hour.
4. Spoon into 2 x 450 g (1 lb) or 1 x 900 g (2 lb) prepared loaf tins.
5. Bake at 180°C (350°F) Gas Mark 4 for approximately 1–1^1/$_2$ hours or until firm on top.
6. Remove from tins and leave to cool on a wire rack.
7. Serve warm or cold with butter, cheese and fruit or nut spreads.

Frozen Raspberry Yogurt Cheesecake

SERVES 8

SPONGE BASE
1 large egg
50 g (2 oz) butter
50 g (2 oz) sugar
25 g (1 oz) brown rice flour
25 g (1 oz) ground almonds

FILLING
500 g (1 lb) fresh raspberries
75 g (3 oz) icing sugar
50 ml (2 fl oz) amaretto liqueur
  (almond flavour)
grated rind and juice of 1 lime
250 ml (^{1}/$_2$ pint) double cream
2 x 100 g (4 oz) cartons of
  raspberry yogurt

1. Preheat the oven to 180°C (350°F) Gas Mark 4. Grease and line an 18 cm (7 inch) loose-bottomed round cake tin with greaseproof paper. Beat the sponge ingredients with an electric hand whisk until light and fluffy. Spoon into the prepared tin and bake for 15–28 minutes or until firm to touch. Turn out and cool on a wire rack.
2. Reserve a few raspberries for decoration. Place the remainder in a bowl with 50 g (2 oz) of the icing sugar, the amaretto and lime juice, then set aside for a few minutes. Blend the cream, yogurt, remaining icing sugar and vanilla in a food processor until thickened.
3. Purée raspberries, sugar, amaretto and lime juice in a food processor, then press through a sieve to remove pips. Fold two-thirds into the cream mixture, reserving the rest for the sauce.
4. Line the cake tin with clingfilm, leaving an overhanging edge, and place the sponge inside.
5. Pour in the cream mixture and freeze for 3–4 hours until set. Lift out the cake using the clingfilm and place on a plate. Allow to stand for 1¹/₂ hours before serving with the remaining raspberries and sauce. Sprinkle with icing sugar and decorate with toasted, flaked almonds.

Fig and Almond Pudding

SERVES 3

10 dried figs
350 ml (³/₄ pint) pure apple juice
285 g (10 oz) plain tofu
50 g (2 oz) ground almonds
1 tbsp lemon juice

2 tsp sugar
1 tsp ground cinnamon
1 tsp vanilla extract
1 tbsp slivered almonds

1. Soak the figs in the apple juice in the refrigerator overnight.
2. Combine the figs, apple juice, tofu, lemon juice, sugar, cinnamon and vanilla in a blender and purée for 2–3 minutes until very smooth, occasionally scraping down the sides of the bowl. Stir in the ground almonds until well combined. Scoop into 3 small serving bowls and decorate with the almonds.

Delicious Christmas Pudding   WOBR

SERVES 10

2 eggs, small, lightly beaten
100 g (4 oz) soy cooking
  margarine, melted
100 g (4 oz) alternative
  breadcrumbs (wheat, oats, rye
  and barley free)
50 g (2 oz) soy flour
50 g (2 oz) cornflour
100 g (4 oz) molasses
1 large cooking apple, chopped
1 tsp ground cinnamon
1 tsp ground ginger
1 tsp mixed spice
225 g (8 oz) raisins

100 g (4 oz) sultanas
100 g (4 oz) currants
50 g (2 oz) mixed candied peel
1 carrot, peeled and grated
50 g (2 oz) flaked almonds
finely grated zest of 1 large orange
  and lemon
3 tbsp rum
3 tbsp brandy
3 tbsp port
1 tsp wheatfree baking powder or
  1 tsp cream of tartar
$^{1}/_{2}$ tsp bicarbonate of soda

1. Lightly grease a 1-litre (2-pint) pudding basin, or two 500–600-ml (1-pint) pudding basins.
2. Mix all the ingredients together in a large bowl, then place in the pudding basin.
3. Cover with greaseproof paper and a layer of muslin or cotton. Tie on with string, and bring the sides of the muslin or cotton up and knot to make a handle which will make it easier to lift out of the pressure-cooker when cooked.
4. Pressure-cook the smaller basins for $1^{1}/_{2}$ hours, 2 hours for the larger basin. Serve with brandy butter.

BREAD AND CAKES

Buckwheat and Rice Bread   WOBR

MAKES 2 LOAVES

This makes brown bread which is crisp on the outside and soft on the inside.

350 g (12 oz) buckwheat flour
175 g (6 oz) brown rice flour
1¹/₂ packets easy-blend yeast
1 tsp sugar

1 tbsp vegetable oil
¹/₂–1 tsp salt
300–350 ml (10–12 fl oz) hand-
    hot water

1. Mix together the flours and the easy-blend yeast.
2. Add the sugar, oil and salt and mix to a thick batter with the hand-hot water.
3. Grease and flour 2 x 450g (1 lb) loaf tins. Divide the mixture between the two tins, cover and leave to rise in a warm place for 20–30 minutes.
4. Bake the loaves in the preheated oven at 230°C (450°F) Gas Mark 8 for 35–40 minutes. The bread will slightly contract from the side of the tins when it is cooked.
5. Cool for 5 minutes in the tins and then turn out on to a wire rack. Slice when cold.

Soy and Buckwheat Loaf   WOBR

150 g (5 oz) buckwheat flour
150 g (5 oz) soy flour
50 g (2 oz) ground almonds
100 g (4 oz) rice flour
15 g (¹/₂ oz) dahl (chickpea) flour
1 tsp bicarbonate of soda
2 tsp baking powder (wheat-free)

1 tsp sugar (optional)
1 tsp salt
20 g (³/₄ oz) butter/2 tbsp oil
1 large egg, beaten
450 ml (15 fl oz) So Good soy
    milk, sheep, goat or cow's milk

1. Heat the oven to 180°C (350°F) Gas Mark 4.
2. Mix the flours together and sift into a large bowl, then mix in the other ingredients. Rub in the butter or pour in the oil, then stir in the beaten egg and milk, making certain that the mixture is thoroughly combined.

3. Grease and line a 1 kg (2 lb) loaf tin or round cake tin and pour in the soda bread mixture (this is quite runny). Bake in the centre of the oven for 45–50 minutes, or until a skewer comes out clean.
4. Allow to cool slightly in the tin, covered with a teacloth, then knock carefully onto a cooling rack.
5. Cover with a teacloth and allow to get completely cold before slicing. Serve with organic butter, nut butters or pure fruit spread.

Note: This bread actually slices and does not crumble – it can be used for sandwiches!

Seed Bread

150 g (5oz) soy flour
150 g (5oz) rice flour
75 g (3oz) potato flour
1 tsp bicarbonate of soda
2 tsp cream of tartar
75 g (3oz) sunflower seeds

50 g (2oz) sesame seeds
50 g (2oz) golden linseeds
50 g (2oz) caraway seeds
310 ml ($^3/_4$ pint) So Good
  soy milk
2 tsp honey

1. Sift flours, cream of tartar and bicarbonate of soda into a large bowl.
2. Add seeds to flour. Mix the honey and So Good and stir into the dry ingredients.
3. Pour mixture into a greased 450-g (1-lb) loaf tin and bake at 180°C (350°F) Gas Mark 4 for 40–50 minutes, or until the sides of the bread come away from the tin.

Potato Shortbread   WOBR

MAKES 8 SLICES

175 g (6 oz) potato flour
100 g (4 oz) margarine

50 g (2 oz) sugar
75 g (3 oz) ground almonds

1. Put all the ingredients into a food processor and beat together for 5–6 seconds. Scrape the bowl and repeat the process until a ball of dough is formed.
2. Put the dough in a greased 17.5–20 cm (7–8 inch) round sandwich tin and press down evenly.
3. Mark out portions with a knife, prick all over and bake in the pre-heated oven at 180°C (350°F) Gas Mark 4 for 35–40 minutes.
4. Cut into wedges and leave to cool in the tin.

Honey Cake

SERVES 12

6 medium eggs
100 g (4 oz) soft brown sugar
185 g (6 oz) clear honey
225 g (8 oz) ground almonds
1 heaped tbsp ground cinnamon
3 tsp ground ginger

3 tsp mixed spice
30 ginger drops (ginger in oil from
the health-food shop)
4 tbsp rice flour
2 tbsp baking powder

1. Beat the eggs until pale and frothy.
2. Melt the sugar and the honey until warmed, then stir in the ground almonds.
3. Add the cinnamon, ginger drops, ground ginger and mixed spice and mix thoroughly with the beaten egg mixture.
4. Fold in the rice flour and add the baking powder. Combine thoroughly and pour into a greased 20 x 35-cm (8 x 14-inch) baking tin. Decorate with almond halves or split almonds and bake for 1 hour.
5. This cake moistens with age, and is great with soy custard or bio yogurt.

Apple and Cinnamon Cake   WOBR

MAKES 8 GOOD-SIZED SLICES

4 large cooking apples
100 g (4oz) brown rice flour
4 large eggs
100 g (4oz) ground almonds
100 g (4oz) caster sugar
100 g (4oz) soft margarine

a few drops of almond essence
1 tbsp ground cinnamon
GARNISH
about 16 apple slices
$^1/_2$ tbsp ground cinnamon
1 tbsp caster sugar

1. Grease a deep 20-cm (8-inch) loose-bottomed circular cake tin. Preheat the oven to 150°C (300°F) Gas Mark 2.
2. Peel, core and slice the apples and leave to soak in cold water.
3. Place the flour, eggs, ground almonds, caster sugar, margarine and almond essence in the bowl of a mixer and beat until light and fluffy.
4. Line the cake tin with approximately 3.75 cm (1$^1/_2$ inch) of mixture. Place most of the garnish apples in the tin and sprinkle with cinnamon and sugar. Spread the additional mixture on the top of the apples and smooth off the top ready for decoration.
5. Gently push the remaining apple slices into the top of the cake in a circle and sprinkle with cinnamon and sugar.
6. Bake in the preheated oven for at least 1 hour until cooked through.

Cool briefly, then gently ease the cake out of the tin and onto a plate.

7. Serve hot as a pudding or cold as a cake with whipped or pouring cream.

Lemon and Almond Cake   WOBR

MAKES ABOUT 8–10 SLICES

175 g (6oz) soft butter
175 g (6oz) caster sugar
3 eggs
175 g (6oz) self-raising flour or
  brown rice flour
150 g (5oz) ground almonds

finely grated rind and juice of
  1 lemon
$^1/_2$ tsp almond essence
TO FINISH
2 lemons
2 tbsp clear honey

1. Preheat the oven to 160°C (325°F) Gas Mark 3. Grease and base line a 20-cm (8-inch) loose-bottomed round cake tin.
2. Place all the cake ingredients in a large bowl. Mix well and beat with a wooden spoon or electric whisk for 2–3 minutes until light and fluffy.
3. Turn the mixture into the prepared cake tin and smooth the top.
4. To finish, pare the rind thinly from the 2 lemons, avoiding the pith, then slice into thin shreds and place on top of the cake.
5. Bake in the preheated oven for 50–60 minutes until golden and firm. Cool in the tin for 10 minutes, then release the sides and remove the cake. Cool on a wire rack.
6. Warm the honey, brush over the top of the cake, and serve.

Ginger Cake   WOBR

MAKES 8 GENEROUS SLICES

100 g (4oz) margarine
75 g (3oz) dark muscovado sugar
150 ml ($^1/_4$ pint) golden syrup
150 ml ($^1/_4$ pint) black treacle
2 tsp ground ginger
$^1/_2$ tsp mixed spice

$^1/_2$–1 tsp baking powder
50 g (2 oz) maize meal
100 (4 oz) potato flour
75 g (3 oz) rice flour
2 eggs, medium
150 ml ($^1/_4$ pint) So Good soy milk

1. Grease a 20-cm (8-inch) round cake tin. Preheat the oven to 160°C (325°F) Gas Mark 3.
2. Melt the margarine, sugar, syrup and treacle together gently, then stir in the ginger and mixed spice.

3. Sift the baking powder and three flours together into a bowl, and make a well in the centre.
4. Add the syrup mixture to the well, and beat until smooth.
5. Lightly beat eggs and milk together, then gradually beat them into the batter.
6. Pour the batter into the prepared tin and bake in the preheated oven for 1 hour. Cool on a cake rack. Add icing if wanted.

Almond Macaroons   WOBR

MAKES 18

2 large egg whites   75 g (3oz) caster sugar
175 g (6oz) ground almonds   18 almond halves

1. Put the unbeaten egg whites into a bowl with the ground almonds and beat well, adding the caster sugar 1 tablespoon at a time.
2. Line biscuit trays with greaseproof paper. With moist hands roll the mixture into balls and flatten with the palm of your hand.
3. Lay the flattened biscuits carefully onto the trays and place an almond half in the middle of each biscuit.
4. Bake in the oven preheated at 180°C (350°F) Gas Mark 4 for 25 minutes or until golden brown.
5. Keep in an airtight tin or freeze.

Coconut Pyramids   WOBR

MAKES ABOUT 24

4 egg yolks or 2 whole eggs   juice and rind of ¹/₂ lemon
75 g (3oz) caster sugar   225 g (8oz) desiccated coconut

1. Beat the egg yolks and sugar together until creamy.
2. Stir in the lemon juice, rind and coconut.
3. Form into pyramid shapes either with your hands or using a moist egg cup and place on a greased baking tray.
4. Bake in the preheated oven at 190°C (375°F) Gas Mark 5 until the tips are golden brown.
5. Keep in an airtight tin or freeze.

POSTSCRIPT

As we now live on average to the ripe old age of 83, there is still a lot of living to be done. If you think of the average lifespan in terms of the months of the year, you are, roughly speaking, currently experiencing 'the summer of your life'. Put in those terms it doesn't sound so bad. Although you may have had your share of 'cloudy' days, the chances are that you will soon emerge from the tunnel, feeling healthier, mentally stronger and physically fitter than you have for years.

Life is about give and take – no doubt you have come to realise that by now – and the same applies at the time of the menopause. There are swings and roundabouts; and what you lose on the youth and beauty stakes you gain with the wisdom of your years and in terms of freedom.

Going through 'the change' is nature's way of helping you to adjust, both physically and mentally. Time always allows us to acclimatise to changes. The menopause is a time for reflection and consideration of what you intend to do with the rest of your life. Having dedicated yourself to others' needs, both at home and at work, it may feel somewhat unrealistic suddenly to think about your own. Well, it is the 'change', isn't it?

These are *your* years and they stretch out before you. This is new territory for women and it's up to you to set the scene both for yourself and for future generations. You can now contemplate your future with optimistic expectation. You need to give considerable thought to what you would like to achieve. Many options will present themselves, bringing with them new horizons. At the time of the menopause, after careful evaluation, women boldly make changes: they go back to college to study subjects they had never dreamed about, they make work and lifestyle changes, become volunteers or start new careers. The common denominator is that they have all focused on a direction that appeals to them, rather than going through the motions to please others. These are years of new-found freedom and independence: your future is what you make it.

If you choose a 'natural' menopause, you will undoubtedly feel that you are in the driving seat. As a result, you will feel a great sense of achievement for having made the journey without swallowing remedies from the pharmaceutical industry. But it's your menopause and it's up to you to decide whether you want to help yourself by following the natural approach or whether you want a little extra hormonal help in the short-term.

In our experience, postmenopausal women become a force to be reckoned with. With new strength and spirit they unknowingly become respected and admired 'towers' in society. They manage to find themselves again after years of being absent. Be as positive as you can while you are making your voyage. Make time for regular rest, relaxation, exercise and, most of all, time to reflect about what you are aiming for in life. If you are in good physical and spiritual shape, the world is your oyster.

Good luck.

APPENDICES

1

FURTHER HELP AND TELEPHONE ADVICE LINES

If you would like to attend one of the WNAS clinics or need further details about our telephone and postal courses of treatment, you can write to the WNAS at the address below with a large self-addressed envelope and four separate first-class stamps. Please state clearly that you require information about our menopause services, as we help women with all sorts of other problems.

I should also be interested to hear about your success using the recommendations in this book.

The address to write to is:

Women's Nutritional Advisory Service
PO Box 268
Lewes
East Sussex BN7 2QN
website http://www.wnas.org
e-mail wnas@wnas.org.uk

All clinic appointments are booked on 01273–487366.

We also have a number of advice lines you may be interested in listening to:

Overcome Menopause Naturally	09062 556602
The Menopause Diet Line	09062 556603
Overcome PMS Naturally	09062 556600
The PMS Diet Line	09062 556601
Beat Sugar Craving	09062 556604
The Vitality Diet Line	09062 556605
Overcoming Breast Tenderness	09062 556606
Overcome Period Pains Naturally	09062 556607
Get Fit for Pregnancy and Breastfeeding	09062 556608
Skin, Nail & Hair Signs of Deficiency	09062 556609

Improve Libido Naturally	09062 556610
Beat Irritable Bowel Syndrome	09062 556611
Overcome Fatigue	09062 556612
Beat Migraine Naturally	09062 556613
Overcome Ovulation Pain	09062 556614
Preventing Osteoporosis	09602 556644
Self-help for Preventing Arthritis	09062 556645
Addressing Heart Disease Naturally	09062 556646
Overcome Constipation Naturally	09062 556647
Detecting and Dealing with Allergies	09062 556648
Directory Helpline	09062 556615

2
DICTIONARY OF TERMS

ABBREVIATIONS
g = gram, mg = milligram (1000 mg = 1g), mcg = microgram (1000 mcg = 1 mg), IU = international unit, kj = kilojoule

Abdomen The cavity between the lower ribs and pelvis in which the ovaries and womb are contained

Acute A term applied to a disease with a rapid onset or brief duration

Adrenal glands The adrenal glands are two small glands situated at the top of the kidneys. They produce several different hormones, most of which are steroid hormones. Hormones from the adrenal glands influence the metabolism of sugar, salt and water and several other functions

Aldactone This is a diuretic drug which helps fluid retention. It inhibits the action of aldosterone, a hormone from the adrenal glands. It is also known as spironolactone

Aldosterone This is a steroid hormone produced by the adrenal glands which is involved in salt and water balance. When it is produced in excess it causes the body to hold water and sodium salt

Allergy An unusual and unexpected sensitivity to a particular substance which causes an adverse reaction. Foods, chemicals and environmental pollutants are common irritants and they may cause a whole range of symptoms including headaches, abdominal bloating and discomfort, skin rashes, eczema and asthma

Antibody A specific form of blood protein able to counteract the effects of bacterial antigens or toxins

Amenorrhoea A complete absence of periods

Amino acids Chains of building blocks which combine together to form the proteins that make living things. There are some 20 or more amino acids, some essential, some non-essential

Antidepressants These are drugs used to suppress symptoms of depression

Biochanin A more recently discovered isoflavone found in the herb Red Clover, chickpeas, lentils and mung beans, biochanin is known to lower blood fats

Bone mineral density Measurement of the mineral density of the bone, usually the neck of the femur or a lumbar vertebra (bone inside back) using specialised X-rays. It is an important assessment of the bone strength and likelihood of fracture

Cancer A general term to describe malignant growths in tissue, which are not encapsulated but infiltrate into surrounding tissue

Candida albicans A yeast-like fungus occurring in moist areas of the body such as the skin folds, mouth, respiratory tract and vagina

Carbohydrates Carbohydrates are the main source of calories (kjs) in almost all diets. Complex carbohydrates are essential nutrients and occur in the form of fruits, vegetables, pulses and grains. They are important energy-giving foods. There are two sorts of complex carbohydrates: the first are digestible, such as the starches, and the second are not digestible and are more commonly known as 'fibre'

Carbohydrates (refined) These consist of foods that have been processed and refined. In the process, white or brown sugar and white flour have had many of the vitamins and minerals present in the original plant removed.

Cardiovascular system The heart, blood vessels and circulation of blood round the body

Cervix The neck of the womb which projects downwards into the vagina

Cholesterol A fat present in the blood and tissues used in the production of all sex hormones. An excess from the diet or metabolism contributes to the risk of heart disease.

Climacteric The menopausal period in women

Collagen A protein that is the principal constituent of white fibrous connective tissue and is present in bone as the framework on which the minerals are arranged

Conjugated oestrogens Oestrogens in their natural, non-synthetic state are teamed up with other components and are termed conjugated oestrogens

Contraceptive An item or method used to prevent pregnancy

Corpus luteum Literally, a little yellow gland or body. It is the part of the ovary that remains after the egg has left. It produces two hormones – oestrogen and progesterone – during the second half of the menstrual cycle

Cyst A sac or cavity containing liquid or semi-solid matter

Cystitis Inflammation of the lining of the bladder which often causes pain and the need to urinate frequently

Daidzein The second major isoflavone to be discovered, daidzein is found predominantly in pulses and acts as an anti-cancer agent. Daidzein is also particularly involved in bone health and may slow bone loss

Deficiency A lack of an essential substance like a vitamin

Diagnosis Process of determining the nature of a disease

Discharge A substance released from the body

Disease A set of signs and symptoms with a definite pathological process

Diuretics Drugs which cause an increased production of urine by the kidneys. They are used to treat fluid retention

Dopamine A brain chemical which affects mood and has a sedating effect

Dysmenorrhoea Painful periods

Endocrine glands Glands that secrete hormones and regulate other organs in the body. The thyroid and the pituitary are endocrine glands

Endometriosis A condition in which the lining of the uterus begins to grow outside the uterus in the abdominal cavity. It is usually a painful condition and can cause infertility

Endometrial cancer Cancer of the lining of the womb. It can occur if the endometrium is overstimulated by some hormones

Endorphins Hormones from the pituitary gland and fluid in the spine which are believed to help control moods, behaviour and part of the workings of the pituitary itself. They may also have an effect on how sugar is used in the body and on other amounts of hormones released from the pituitary gland and the ovaries. If this is so, the production of oestrogen and progesterone could be affected by endorphins

Essential fatty acids One of the essential groups of foods which we need to remain healthy. These are essential fats that are necessary for normal cell structure and body function. There are two: linoleic and linolenic acids. They are called 'essential' because they cannot be made by the body but have to be eaten in the diet

Fertilisation The impregnation of the female sex cell by a male sex cell

Fibroids A benign tumour of fibrous and muscular tissue which often develops in the womb

Follicle Stimulating Hormone (FSH) A hormone of the pituitary gland which stimulates the growth of the follicles in the ovaries

Follicular phase The first half of the menstrual cycle when an egg is growing in the ovary. The egg is surrounded by cells which produce the hormone oestrogen and which thus prepare the uterus for conception. The egg and surrounding cells are called a follicle

Formononetin A more recently discovered isoflavone, formononetin is found in the herb Red Clover, chickpeas, lentils and mung beans

Genistein The most extensively studied isoflavone to date, genistein acts as an anti-oestrogen in a similar way to the drug Tamoxifen administered for breast cancer but without the side-effects

Glucose A form of sugar found in the diet or released by the liver into the blood-stream which is then used by the brain for energy. This is the only source of energy it can use

Graafian follicle A mature egg which is surrounded by a bag of fluid within the ovary

Gynaecologist A person who specialises in diseases and problems of the female reproductive system

Heart attack Sudden damage to the heart muscle due to a blockage in its supply of blood. Sudden severe pains in the chest and possibly arms result. Also known as a coronary thrombosis or myocardial infarction

Hormonal implant A substance inserted into the body

Hormone Replacement Therapy (HRT) Hormones used to treat females suffering symptoms relating to the menopause

Hormones Substances formed chiefly in the endocrine glands which then enter the blood-stream and control the activity of an organ or body function. Adrenalin and insulin are hormones, as are oestrogen and progesterone

Hot flush A sudden feeling of warmth and usually perspiration of the skin of the face and neck

Hyperhydration – too much water present A term used to describe water retention in the body

Hypoglycaemia – low blood sugar A condition in which there is a deficiency of insulin or lack of food. As glucose is required for normal brain function, mental disturbance can occur, as can other symptoms: headaches, weakness, faintness, irritability, palpitations, mood swings, sweating and hunger. One of the most common contributing factors is an excess of refined carbohydrates in the diet

Hypothalamus The region of the brain controlling temperature, hunger, thirst and the hormones produced by the pituitary gland

Hysterectomy A surgical procedure to remove the womb and the Fallopian tubes. Sometimes one or both ovaries are also removed

Immunology The study of the body's immunity to disease

Incontinence Involuntary lack of control in passing urine

Infertility Inability for a woman or a man to be able to reproduce

Inflammation The body's protective response to infection or injury which results in pain, swelling and heat of the affected part

Insomnia Inability to sleep

Isoflavones Found mainly in legumes and pulses, isoflavones are best known for their effects on oestrogen metabolism and female health

Lignans Found mainly in wheat bran and linseeds, lignans are converted by bacteria in the gut into a number of hormone-like compounds which are believed to lower the risk of certain cancers, particularly breast cancer.

Luteal phase The time after the egg has left the follicle in the ovary and the follicle then becomes a gland known as the corpus luteum. The corpus luteum mainly produces progesterone

Luteinizing Hormone (LH) The pituitary hormone that fosters the development of the corpus luteum

Mastectomy Surgical removal of a breast

Menarche The start of menstruation

Menopause The time at which the last natural period takes place. It is a date, not several months or years

Menstruation The monthly discharge of blood from the uterus

Menorrhagia An excessive loss of blood during each period

Menses The discharge of blood and tissue lining from the uterus which occurs approximately every four weeks between puberty and the menopause

Menstrual cycle The monthly cycle involving the pituitary gland, ovaries and uterus in which an egg is produced ready for conception. In each cycle an egg in the ovary is released and the lining of the womb develops ready for conception and implantation of the fertilised egg. If this does not occur, the lining of the womb is shed and a period occurs

Menstrual symptomatology diary A chart which is a daily record of all symptoms that occur throughout the menstrual cycle

Metabolism The process by which the body maintains life. It is the cycle of nutrients being broken down to produce energy which is then used by the body to build new cells and tissues, provide heat, growth and physical activity. The metabolic rate tends to vary from person to person, depending on their age, sex and lifestyle

Mittelschmerz Pain associated with ovulation which usually occurs about halfway through the menstrual cycle. Translated, it means 'middle pain'

Nutrition The British Society for Nutritional Medicine's definition is the 'sum of the processes involved in taking nutrients, assimilating and utilising them'. In other words, the quality of the diet and the ability of your body to utilise the individual nutrients and so maintain health

Oestrogen A steroid hormone produced in large quantities by the ovaries and in smaller amounts by the adrenal glands. It's responsible at puberty for the development of breasts and other sexual characteristics. Oestrogen is also responsible for the production of fertile cervical mucus, the opening of the cervix and the building-up of blood in the lining of the uterus as it prepares for a fertilised egg

Omega-3 fatty acids Essential fatty acids found mainly in oily fish and some vegetable oils

Omega-6 fatty acid Essential fatty acid found in some vegetable oils. Commonest type known as linoleic acid. Evening primrose oil contains a very specialized omega-6 essential fatty acid

Oophorectomy Surgical removal of an ovary

Oral contraceptives Medication taken orally to prevent pregnancy

Osteoporosis Thinning of the bones which leads to their brittleness and weakness

Ovaries A pair of glands on either side of the uterus in which eggs and sex hormones, including oestrogen, are produced

Ovulation The release of the ripe egg (ovum) from the ovary. The two ovaries ovulate alternately every month. Occasionally, the two ovaries ovulate simultaneously, in which case the result may be twins

Ovum The egg which is released from the ovary at the time of ovulation

Palpitations The heart beating too fast and sometimes irregularly

Pelvic Inflammatory Disease (PID) Inflammation or infection of the internal female genital organs

Perimenopausal The time around the menopause especially the time leading up to it

Phytates Until recently, phytic acid (derived from phytates) was considered to be a substance to be avoided because of its ability to impede the absorption of important minerals. However, more recent research suggests that it has beneficial antioxidant properties

Phytochemicals These are chemicals in plants which have antioxidant/anti-cancer properties

Phytoestrogens These are a family of naturally occuring substances with a chemical structure very similar to our own female hormone oestrogen

Phytosterols These have been shown to inhibit the development of cancers, including colon and skin cancer, and may also help to prevent heart disease by helping to control cholesterol levels

Pituitary gland A small gland situated at the base of the brain which produces many hormones, among which are those that stimulate the ovaries and thyroid

Postmenopause This refers to the time after the menopause

Premenstrual A term used to describe the time before the arrival of a period

Premenstrual syndrome A collection of mental and physical symptoms that can manifest themselves before the onset of a period

Premenstrual tension The name first given in 1931 by Dr Frank to the physical and mental symptoms detected before a period. Today the correct name is premenstrual syndrome. However, many women still prefer to call the condition PMT – premenstrual tension

Progesterone A hormone secreted by the corpus luteum of the ovary during the second half of the menstrual cycle. Progesterone is an important hormone during pregnancy

Progestogens A group of synthetic hormones with actions similar to progesterone

Prolactin The hormone involved in milk production which is secreted by the pituitary gland. It is also known to affect the water and mineral balance in the body and in some women it may play a part in premenstrual changes

Prostaglandins Hormone-like substances found in almost every cell in the body. They are necessary for the normal function of involuntary muscles, including the heart, the uterus, blood vessels, the lungs and the intestines. Sometimes regarded as health-controllers, as they seem to play an important part in controlling many essential body functions. They do not come directly from the diet, but are made in the body itself, so the body relies on a good diet in order to produce them. The special substances the body needs to make prostaglandins are called **essential fatty acids**

Puberty The age at which the male and female reproductive organs begin to function

Saponins Like phytates, saponins have antioxidant properties that protect us from the damaging effects of free radicals as well as helping to control cholesterol

Serotonin A brain chemical that influences mood

Serum A clear fluid residue of blood

Sterilisation A surgical procedure rendering males and females infertile

Steroids Substances which have a particular chemical structure in common. All the sex hormones, such as oestrogen, progesterone and testosterone are steroids. The term 'steroid' is also used in the context of corticosteroids (or cortisone), powerful agents that suppress inflammation and allergic reactions

Symptom An indication of disease such as a feeling, pain or complaint felt by the patient

Testosterone The male sex hormone

Thyroid gland A gland in the neck which produces the hormone thyroxine. The thyroid gland regulates the metabolism

Tranquillisers A group of drugs which artificially sedate the body. They can be useful in the short-term but in the long-term they may have addictive qualities

Urethra The canal through which urine is released from the bladder

Uterus (womb) A sac-like organ located in the abdomen of a woman and designed to hold and nourish a growing child from conception until birth

Vagina The passage that leads from the uterus to the external genital organs

Virus A microscopic organism capable of producing infection

Vulva External female genital organs

Withdrawal bleed This bleed occurs when the lining of the womb is lost as a result of withdrawal of oestrogen. This is a dependable response by the womb, and will almost always occur unless the woman is pregnant

Womb The uterus. It is situated at the top of the vagina and receives the eggs, where they can develop into a pregnancy if fertilised

Xenoestrogens These are derived from chemicals, primarily DDT, PCBs, dioxins and fungicides, and the contraceptive pill. They interact with the receptor sites within a cell, but they block normal hormone activity

3
RECOMMENDED READING

Note
UK, USA and A denote the following books are available in Great Britain, the United States of America and Australia.

General health

1. *Nutritional Medicine*
   by Dr Stephen Davies and Dr Alan Stewart
   (published by Pan Books) UK A
2. *The Holistic Approach to Cancer*
   by Ian C.B. Pearce
   (published by The C.W. Daniel Co. Ltd) UK USA
3. *Getting Sober and Loving It*
   by Joan and Derek Taylor
   (published by Vermilion) UK A
4. *Tired all the Time*
   by Dr Alan Stewart
   (published by Vermilion) UK USA A
5. *Memory Power*
   by Ursula Markham
   (published by Vermilion) UK A
6. *Alternative Health Aromatherapy*
   by Gill Martin
   (published by Optima) UK USA A
7. *Alternative Health Acupuncture*
   by Dr Michael Nightingale
   (published by Optima) UK USA A
8. *Alternative Health Osteopathy*
   by Stephen Sandler
   (published by Optima) UK USA

9. *Bone Boosters – Natural Ways to Beat Osteoporosis*
   by Diana Moran and Helen Franks
   (published by Boxtree) UK
10. *No More IBS!*
   by Maryon Stewart and Dr Alan Stewart
   (published by Vermilion) UK A
11. *Natural Health Bible*
   by Maryon Stewart and Dr Alan Stewart
   (published by Vermilion) UK A
12. *No More PMS!*
   by Maryon Stewart
   (published by Vermilion) UK A
13. *Beat PMS Cookbook*
   by Maryon Stewart
   (available from the WNAS) UK
14. *Beat Sugar Craving*
   by Maryon Stewart
   (available from the WNAS) UK
15. *Understanding Cystitis*
   by Angela Kilmartin
   (published by Arrow Books) UK A
16. *The Book of Massage*
   by Lucy Lidell
   (published by Ebury Press) UK
17. *Candida Albicans*
   by Gill Jacobs
   (published by Optima) UK USA A
18. *Escape from Tranquillisers and Sleeping Pills*
   by Larry Nield
   (published by Ebury Press) UK
19. *Alternative Health for Women*
   by Patsy Wescott
   (published by Thorsons) UK
20. *The Women's Guide to Homoeopathy, The Natural Way to a Healthier Life for Women*
   by Dr Andrew Lockie and Dr Nicola Geddes
   (published by Hamish Hamilton) UK
21. *The Well Woman's Self-Help Book*
   by Nikki Bradford
   (published by Sidgwick & Jackson) UK

22. *Food Irradiation: The Facts*
    by Tony Webb and Dr Tim Lang
    (published by Thorsons) UK
23. *Candida – Diet Against It*
    by Luc de Schepper
    (published by Foulsham) UK
24. *Coming Off Tranquillisers*
    by Dr Shirley Trickett
    (published by Thorsons) UK USA
    (Lothian Publishing Company) A
25. *Osteoporosis*
    by Kathleen Mayes
    (published by Thorsons) UK
26. *Natural Hormone Health*
    by Arabella Melville
    (published by Thorsons) UK USA A
27. *Fibromyalgia and Muscle Pain*
    by Leon Chaitow
    (published by Thorsons) UK
28. *Alexander Technique*
    by Chris Stevens
    (published by Random House) UK
29. *Evening Primrose Oil*
    by Judy Graham
    (published by Thorsons) UK
30. *A Guide to Herbal Remedies*
    by Mark Evans
    (published by The C. W. Daniel Co. Ltd) UK USA
31. *Hysterectomy – New Options and Advances*
    by Lorraine Dennerstein, Carl Wood and Ann Westmore,
    2nd edition (published by Oxford University Press, Melbourne)
    UK A
32. *Easy Way to Stop Smoking*
    by Allen Carr
    (published by Penguin) UK
33. *The Phyto Factor*
    by Maryon Stewart
    (published by Vermilion) UK A
34. *Maryon Stewart's Zest for Life Plan*
    (published by Headline) UK A

35. GM FREE A *Shopper's Guide to Genetically Modified Food*
    by Sue Dibb and Dr Tim Lobstein
    (published by Virgin)
36. *Entometriosis – A Key to Healing Through Nutrition*
    by Dian Shepperson Mills & Michael Vernon
    (published by Element Books Ltd)

Diet

1. *The New Why You Didn't Need Meat*
   by Peter Cox
   (published by Bloomsbury) UK A
2. *Organic Consumer Guide/Food You Can Trust*
   edited by David Mabey and Alan and Jackie Gear
   (published by Thorsons) UK
3. *The New Raw Energy*
   by Leslie and Susannah Kenton
   (published by Vermilion) UK
   (Doubleday) A

Stress

1. *Aromatherapy for Women and Children*
   by Jane Dye
   (published by The C. W. Daniel Co. Ltd) UK USA
2. *Stress Wise*
   by Dr Terry Looker and Dr Olga Gregson
   (published by Headway) UK
3. *Tranquillisation: The Non-Addictive Way*
   by Phyllis Speight
   (published by The C. W. Daniel Co. Ltd) UK USA

Recipe Books

1. *The Single Vegan*
   by Leah Leneman
   (published by Thorsons) UK
2. *The Complete Low-Fat Cookbook*
   by Sue Kreitzman
   (published by Piatkus) UK
3. *Everyday Wheat and Gluten-Free Cookery Book*
   by Michelle Berrydale

4. *Dove's Farm Gluten-free Baking*
5. *The Stamp Collection Cookbook*
   by Terence Stamp and Elizabeth Buxton
   (published by Ebury Press) UK

Drugs

1. *What Do You Know About Drugs?*
   by Sanders and Myers
   (published by Gloucester Press) UK
2. *Forbidden Drugs – Understanding Drugs and How People Take Them*
   by P. Robson
   (published by Oxford University Press) UK

Exercise

1. *The Y's Way to Physical Fitness*
   by Clayton R. Myers and Lawrence A. Golding
   (available from YMCA) UK
2. *YMCA Guide to Exercise to Music*
   by Rodney Cullum and Lesley Mowbray
   (available from YMCA) UK
3. *Pilates – The Way Forward*
   by Lynne Robinson and Gordon Thompson
   (published by Pan) UK

Pregnancy

1. *Healthy Parents, Healthy Baby*
   by Maryon Stewart
   (published by Headline) UK A

4
USEFUL ADDRESSES

UK
Action against Allergy
PO Box 278
Twickenham TW1 4QQ

Age Concern
Astral House
1268 London Road
London SW16 4ER
Tel: 020 8679 8000

Alcoholics Anonymous (AA)
General Services Office
PO Box 1
Stonebow House
Stonebow
York YO1 2NJ
Tel: 01904 644026

Amarant Trust
11–13 Charter House Buildings
London EC1M 7AN
Tel: 01293 413000

*ASH (Campaign for Freedom
from Tobacco)*
Devon House
12–15 Dartmouth Street
London SW1H 9BL
Tel: 020 7314 1360

*British Acupuncture Register and
Directory*
34 Alderney Street
London SW1V 4EU
Tel: 020 7834 1012

British Allergy Foundation
Deepdene House
30 Bellegrove Road
Welling
Kent DA16 3BY
Tel: 020 8303 8525
Helpline: 020 8303 8583
(10–3, weekdays)

British Association for Counselling
1 Regent Place
Rugby
Warwickshire CV21 2PJ
Tel: 01788 578328 (info)

*British College of Naturopathy and
Osteopathy*
6 Netherhall Gardens
London NW3 5RR
Tel: 020 7435 6464

*The British Homoeopathic
Association*
27a Devonshire Street
London W1N 1RJ
Tel: 020 7935 2163

British Hypnotherapy Association
67 Upper Berkeley Street
London W1H 7DH
Tel: 020 7723 4443

British Osteopathic Association Clinic
8–10 Boston Place
London NW1 6QH
Tel: 020 7262 1128

British School of Osteopathy
Administration and Clinics
1–4 Suffolk Street
London SW1Y 4HG
Tel: 020 7930 9254

British Wheel of Yoga
1 Hamilton Place
Boston Road
Sleaford
Lincolnshire NG34 7ES
Tel: 01529 306851

CAN (Northamptonshire Council
    on Addiction)
81 St Giles Street
Northampton NN1 1JF
Tel: 01604 22121

Chiropractic Patients Association
8 Centre One
Lysander Way
Old Sarum Park
Salisbury
Wiltshire SP4 6BU
Tel: 01722 416027

The Council for Acupuncture
206–208 Latimer Road
London W10 2RE
Tel: 020 8964 0222

Depression Alliance
PO Box 1022
London SE1 7QB
Tel: 020 7721 7672

Eating Disorders Association
First Floor
Wensum House
103 Prince of Wales Road
Norwich NR1 1DW
Tel: 01603 619090

The European School of Osteopathy
104 Tonbridge Road
Maidstone
Kent ME16 8SL
Tel: 01622 671558

Exercise Association
Unit 4, Angel Gate
City Road
London EC1V 2PT
Tel: 020 7278 0811

The Faculty of Homoeopathy
The Royal London Homoeopathic
    Hospital
Hahnemann House
2 Powis Place
Great Ormond Street
London WC1N 3HT
Tel: 020 7837 3091, Ext. 72/85

Friends of the Earth
26–28 Underwood Street
London N1 7JQ
Tel: 020 7490 1555

The Henry Doubleday Research
    Association
Ryton Gardens
National Centre for Organic
    Gardening
Ryton on Dunsmore
Coventry CV8 3LG
Tel: 01203 303517

Homoeopathic Development
    Foundation
19a Cavendish Square
London W1M 9AD
Tel: 020 7629 3205

Migraine Trust
45 Great Ormond Street
London WC1N 3HZ
Tel: 020 7278 2676

The National Endometriosis Society
Suite 50, Westminster Palace
   Gardens
1–7 Artillery Road
London SW1R 1RL
Tel: 020 7222 2776

The National Institute of Medical
   Herbalists
56 Longbrook Street
Exeter EX4 6AH
Tel: 01392 426022

The National Osteoporosis Society
Barton Meade House
PO Box 10
Radstock
Bath BA3 3YB

National Society for Research into
   Allergy
PO Box 45
Hinckley
Leicestershire LE10 1JY
Tel: 01455 851546

Patients' Association
8 Guildford Street
London WC1N 1DT
Tel: 020 7242 3460

Positively Women
347–349 City Road
London EC1V 1LR
Tel: 020 7713 0222

Release
388 Old Street
London EC1V 9LT
Tel: 020 7729 9904

The Samaritans
10 The Grove
Slough SL1 1QP
Tel: 01753 532713

School of Phytotherapy (Herbal
   Medicine)
Bucksteep Manor
Bodle Street Green
Nr. Hailsham BN27 4RJ
Tel: 01323 833812/4

The Shiatsu Society
31 Pullman Lane
Godalming
Surrey GU7 1XY
Tel: 01483 860 771

Society for the Promotion of
   Nutritional Therapy (SPNT)
PO Box 626
Woking GU22 0XD
Tel: 01483 740903

The Soil Association
86–88 Colston Street
Bristol BS1 5BB
Tel: 01272 290661

The Sports Council
16 Upper Woburn Place
London WC1H 0QP
Tel: 020 7388 1277

Trax (UK) Ltd.
National Tranquilliser Advice
   Centre
Registered Office
25a Masons Avenue
Wealdstone, Harrow
Middlesex HA3 5AH
Tel: (client line) 020 8427 2065
(24 hr answering service 020 8427
   2827)

Vegan Society
Donald Watson House
7 Battle Road
St Leonards-on-Sea
East Sussex TN37 7AA
Tel: 01424 427393

Vegetarian Society
Parkdale
Dunham Road
Altrincham
Cheshire WA14 4QG
Tel: 0161 928 0793

Women's Health
52 Featherstone Street
London EC1Y 8RT
Tel: 020 7251 6580

The Women's Nutritional Advisory
  Service
PO Box 268
Lewes
East Sussex BN7 2QN
Tel: 01273 487366

YMCA
112 Great Russell Street
London WC1B 3NQ
Tel: 020 7637 8131

Australia

Adelaide Women's Community
  Health
64 Pennington Terrace
Nth Adelaide SA 5006
Tel: 08 267 5366

Blackmores Limited – Women's
  Health Advisory Service
23 Roseberry Street
PO Box 258
Balgowlah
NSW 2093
Tel: 02 951 0111

Liverpool Women's Health Centre
26 Bathurst Street
Liverpool
NSW 2170
Tel: 02 601 3555

Women's Health Advisory Service
155 Eaglecreek Road
Werombi 2570
NSW
Tel: 046 531 445

New Zealand

Health Alternative for Women
Room 101, Cranmer Centre
PO Box 884
Christchurch
Tel: 03 796 970

Papakura Women's Centre
4 Opaneke Road
Papakura
Auckland
Tel: 08 267 5366

Tauranga Women's Centre
PO Box 368
Tauranga
Tel: 07 783 530

West Auckland Women's Centre
PO Box 69116
Glendene
Auckland
Tel: 09 838 6381

Women's Health Collective
63 Ponsonby Road
Ponsonby
Auckland
Tel: 09 764 506

5
REFERENCES

2 Set Sail for the Menopause

1. Wilbush, J., 'Climacteric Disorders – Historical Perspectives', in *The Menopause*, Eds. Studd, J.W.W., Whitehead, M.I. Blackwell Scientific Publications, Oxford, 1988, pp 1–14.

3 The Symptoms of the Menopause

1. Ginsburg, J., 'What determines the age at the menopause?' *The British Medical Journal* 1991; 302: 1288–9.
2. Mahadevan, K., Murthy, M.S.R., Reddy, P.R., Bhaskaran, S., 'Early Menopause and its Determinants'. *Journal of Biosocial Science* 1982; 14: 473–9.
3. Magos, A.L., Brewster, E., Singh, R., O'Dowd, T., Brincat, M., Studd, J.W.W., 'The effects of norethisterone in postmenopausal women on oestrogen replacement therapy: a model for the premenstrual syndrome'. *British Journal of Obstetrics and Gynaecology* 1986; 93: 1290–96.
4. Wilcox, L.S. et al, 'Hysterectomy in the United States'. *Obstetrics and Gynecology*, 1994; 83: 549–55.
5. Carlson, K.J., Miller, B.A., Fowler, F.J., 'The Maine Women's Health Study: I. Outcomes of hysterectomy.' *Obstetrics and Gynecology* 1994; 83: 556–65.
6. Guillebaud, J., 'Contraception for women over 35 years of age'. *British Journal of Family Planning* 1992; 17: 115–18.
7. France, K., Schofield, M.J., Lee, C., 'Patterns and correlates of hormone replacement therapy use among middle-aged Australian women'. *Women's Health* 1997; summer: 3(2) 121–38.
8. MacLennan, A.H., Wilson, D.H., Taylor, A.W., 'Hormone replacement therapies in women at risk of cardiovascular disease and osteoporosis in South Australia in 1997'. *Med J Aust* 1999; 170(11): 524–7.
9. Nachtigall, L.B., Nachtigall, M.J., Nachtigall, L.E., 'Nonprescription alternatives to Hormone Replacement Therapy'. *The Female Patient* 1999; 24: 45–50.

4 Medical Risks Following the Menopause
1. Haas, S., Schiff, I., 'Symptoms of Oestrogen Deficiency', in *The Menopause*, Eds. Studd, J.W.W., Whitehead, M.I. Blackwell Scientific Publications, Oxford, 1988, pp 15–23.
2. Sturdee, D., Brincat, M., 'The Hot Flush', in *The Menopause*, Eds. Studd, J.W.W., Whitehead, M.I. Blackwell Scientific Publications, Oxford, 1988, pp 24–42.
3. Brincat, M., Studd, J.W.W., 'Skin and the Menopause', in *The Menopause*, Eds. Studd, J.W.W., Whitehead, M.I. Blackwell Scientific Publications, Oxford, 1988, pp 85–101.
4. Hunter, M., 'Psychological Aspects of the Climacteric and the Postmenopause', in *The Menopause*, Eds. Studd, J.W.W., Whitehead, M.I. Blackwell Scientific Publications, Oxford, 1988, pp 55–64.

5 The Rational Approach to HRT
1. Wilbush, J., 'Climacteric Disorders – Historical Perspectives', in *The Menopause*, Eds. Studd, J.W.W., Whitehead, M.I. Blackwell Scientific Publications, Oxford, 1988, pp 1–14.
2. Wilson, R.C.D., *Understanding HRT and the Menopause*. Consumers Association, London, 1992.

7 Nutrition and Hormone Function
1. Goldin, B.R., Aldercreutz, H., Dwyer, J.T., Swenson, L., Warram, J.H., Gorbach, S.L., 'Effect of diet on excretion of estrogens in pre- and postmenopausal women'. *Cancer Research* 1981; 41: 3771–3.
2. Armstrong, B.K., Brown, J.B., Clarke, H.T., Crooke, D.K., Hahnel, R., Masarei, J.R., Ratajczak, T., 'Diet and reproductive hormones: a study of vegetarian and nonvegetarian postmenopausal women'. *Journal of the National Cancer Institute* 1981; 67: 761–7.
3. Hill, P., Garabaczewski, L., Helman, P., Huskisson, J., Wynder, E.L., 'Diet, lifestyle and menstrual activity'. *American Journal of Nutrition* 1980; 33: 1192–8.
4. Davies, S., Stewart, A., *Nutritional Medicine*, Pan Books, London, 1987.
5. McLaren, H.C., 'Vitamin E and the menopause'. *British Medical Journal* 1949; Dec 17th: 1378–81.
6. Ford, K.A., LaBarbera, A.R., 'Cationic modulation of follicle-stimulating hormone binding to granulosa cell receptor'. *Biology of Reproduction* 1987; 36: 643–50.
7. Feldman, D., Stathis, P.A., Hirst, M.A., Stover, E.P., Do, Y.S., 'Saccharomyces cervisiae produces a yeast substance that exhibits estrogenic activity in mammalian systems'. *Science* 1984; 224: 1109–11.
8. Punnonen, R., Lukola, A., 'Oestrogen-like effect of ginseng'. *British Medical Journal* 1980; 281: 1110.

9. Wilcox, G., Wahlqvist, M.L., Burger, H.G., Medley, G., 'Oestrogenic effects of plant foods in postmenopausal women'. *British Medical Journal* 1990; 301: 905.

10. Van Papendorp, D.H., Coetzer, H., Kruger, M.C., 'Biochemical profile of osteoporotic patients on essential fatty acid supplementation'. *Nutrition Research* 15(3): 325–34.

11. Prior, J.C., 'Progesterone as a bone-trophic hormone.' *Endocrine Reviews* 11(2): 1990; 386–98.

12. Lee, J.R., 'Osteoporosis reversal with transdermal progesterone'. *The Lancet* 1990; 336: 1327.

13. Holt, *Soy for Health – The Definitive Medical Guide*, Mary Ann Liebert, Inc., New York, 1996.

14. Messina, M., Messina, V., *The Simple Soybean and Your Health*, Avery Publishing Group, New York, 1994.

15. Dalais, F.S., Rice, G.E., et al., 'The effects of phyto-oestrogens in postmenopausal women'. Submitted to *Maturitas*, 1997.

16. Murkies, A.L., Lombard, C., Strauss, B.J.G., Wilcox, G., Burger, H.G., Morton, M.S., 'Dietary flour supplementation decreases postmenopausal hot flushes: effect of soy and wheat'. *Maturitas* 1995; 21:189–95.

17. Baird, D.D., Umbach, D.M., Lansdell, L., Hughes, C.L., Setchell, K.D.R., Weinberg, C.R., Haney, A.F., Wilcox, A.J., McLachlan, J.A., 'Dietary intervention study to assess estrogenicity of dietary soy among postmenopausal women'. *Journal of Clinical Endocrinology and Metabolism* 1995; 80:5.

8 The Phytoestrogen Factor

1. St Clair, R.W., 'Estrogens and atheroslclerosis: phytoestrogens and selective estrogen receptor mondulators'. *Curr Opin Lipidol* 1998; 9(5): 457–63.

2. Eden, J. 'Phytoestrogens and the menopause'. *Baillière's Clinical Endocrinology and Metabolism* 1998; 12(4):581–87.

9: Your Continued Good Health

1. MIMS, December, 1996. Haymarket Medical Ltd., London.

2. Jacobs, H.S., Loeffler F.E., 'Postmenopausal hormone replacement therapy'. *British Medical Journal* 1992; 305: 1403–8.

3. Grady, D. et al., 'Hormone therapy to prevent disease and prolong life in postmenopausal women'. *Annals of Internal Medicine* 1992; 117: 1016–37.

4. Stampfer, M.J., et al., 'Postmenopausal estrogen therapy and cardiovascular disease'. *The New England Journal of Medicine* 1991; 325: 756–62.

5. Barret-Connor, E., Bush T.L., 'Estrogen and coronary heart disease in women'. *Journal of the American Medical Association* 1991; 265: 1861–7.

6. Hemminki, E., Sihvo, S., 'A review of postmenopausal Hormone Replacement Therapy recommendations: potential for selection bias'. *Obstetrics and Gynaecology* 1993; 82: 1021–8.

7. Hunt, K., Vessey, M., McPherson, K., 'Mortality in a cohort of long-term users of Hormone Replacement Therapy: an updated analysis'. *British Journal of Obstetrics and Gynaecology* 1990; 97: 1080–86.

8. Nabulsi, A.A., et al., 'Association of Hormone-Replacement Therapy with various cardiovascular risk factors in postmenopausal women'. *The New England Journal of Medicine* 1993; 328: 1069–75.

9. Lindheim, S.R., et al., 'The independent effects of exercise and estrogen on lipids and lipoproteins in postmenopausal women'. *Obstetrics and Gynaecology* 1994; 83: 167–72.

10. Ross, D., Stevenson, J., 'HRT and cardiovascular disease'. *British Journal of Sexual Medicine* 1993; Nov/Dec: 10–13.

11. Rosano, G.M.C., et al., 'Beneficial effect of oestrogen on exercise-induced myocardial ischaemia in women with coronary heart disease'. *The Lancet* 1993; 342: 133–6.

12. Martin, K.A., Freeman, M.W., 'Postmenopausal Hormone-Replacement Therapy'. *The New England Journal of Medicine* 1993; 328: 1115–17.

13. Magos, A.L., Brewster, E., Singh, R., O'Dowd, T., Brincat, M., Studd, J.W.W., 'The effects of norethisterone in postmenopausal women on oestrogen replacement therapy: a model for the premenstrual syndrome'. *British Journal of Obstetrics and Gynaecology* 1986; 93: 1290–96.

14. Coope, J., Thompson, J.M., Poller, L., 'Effects of "natural oestrogen" replacement therapy on menopausal symptoms and blood clotting'. *British Medical Journal* 1975; 4: 139–43.

15. Wallace, W.A., 'Hormone Replacement Therapy and the Surgeon', in *British Menopause Society Newsletter*, December 1993, pp 19–21.

16. Spencer, C., Leyva, F., Stevenson, J., 'Rethinking HRT contraindications'. *British Journal of Sexual Medicine* November/December, 1996; 19–22.

17. Daly, E., Vessey, M.P., Hawkins, M.M., Carson, J.L., Gough, P., Marsh, S., 'Risk of venous thromboembolism in users of hormone replacement therapy'. *The Lancet* 1996; 348: 977–80.

18. Jick, H., Derby, L.E., Myers, M.W., Vasilakis, C., Newton, K.M., 'Risk of hospital admission for idiopathic venous thromboembolism amongst users of postmenopausal oestrogens'. *The Lancet* 1996; 348: 981–3.

19. Grodstein, F., Stampfer, M.J. Golchaber, S.Z., et al., 'Prospective study of exogenous hormones and risk of pulmonary embolism in women'. *The Lancet* 1996; 348: 983-7.

20. Lee Alekel, D., St Germain, A., Peterson, C.T., Hanson, K., Stewart, J.W., Toda, T., 'Isoflavone-rich Soy Protein Isolate Exerts Significant Bone-Sparing in the Lumbar Spine of Perimenopausal Women'. Third

International Symposium on the Role of Soy in Preventing and Treating Chronic Disease, Washington DC 30 Oct–3 Nov, 1999. Abstract.

21. Scheiber, M.D., Liu, J.H., Subbiah, M.T.R., Rebar, R.W., Setchell, K., 'Dietary Soy Isoflavones Favourably Influence Lipids and Bone Turnover in Healthy Postmenopausal Women'. Third International Symposium on the Role of Soy in Preventing and Treating Chronic Disease, Washington DC 30 Oct–3 Nov, 1999. Abstract.

22. Law, M.R., Wald, N.J., Meade, T.W., 'Strategies for the prevention of osteoporosis and hip fracture'. The British Medical Journal 1991; 303: 453–9.

23. Compston, J.E., 'Risk factors for osteoporosis'. Clinical Endocrinology 1992; 36: 223–4.

24. Freudenheim, J.L., Johnson, N.E., Smith, E.L., 'Relationships between usual nutrient intake and bone-mineral content of women 35–65 years of age: longitudinal and cross-sectional analysis'. The American Journal of Clinical Nutrition 1986; 44: 863–76.

25. Kanis, J.A. et al., 'Evidence of efficacy of drugs affecting bone metabolism in preventing hip fracture'. British Medical Journal 1992; 305: 1124–8.

26. Storm, T., Thamsborg, G., Steiniche, T., Genant, H.K., Sorensen, O.H., 'Effect of intermittent cyclical etidronate therapy on bone mass and fracture rate in women with postmenopausal osteoporosis'. The New England Journal of Medicine 1990; 322: 1265–71.

27. LaCroix, A.Z., et al., 'Thiazide diuretic agents and the incidence of hip fracture'. The New England Journal of Medicine 1990; 322: 286–90.

28. Ettinger, B., Grady, D., 'The waning effect of postmenopausal estrogen therapy on osteoporosis'. The New England Journal of Medicine 1993; 329: 1192–3.

29. Recker, R.R., 'Calcium absorption and achlorhydria'. The New England Journal of Medicine 1985; 313: 70–73.

30. Liberman, U. A., et al., 'Effect of oral alendronate on bone mineral density and the incidence of fractures in post menopausal osteoporosis'. The New England Journal of Medicine 1995; 333: 1437-43

31. Black, D. M., Cummings. S. R., et al., 'Randomised trial of effect of alendronate on risk of fracture in women with existing vertebral fractures'. The Lancet 1996; 348: 1535-41.

10 Dining at the Captain's Table – Your Guide to Phytoestrogen-Rich Diet

1. Adlercreutz, H. & Mazur, W. Phyto-oestrogens and Western Diseases. The Finnish Medical Society DUODECIM, Annals of Medicine 1997; 29: 95–120.

2. Mazur, W., Phytoestrogen content in foods. Baillière's Clinical Endocrinology and Metabolism 1998; 12(4): 729–42.

3. Than, D. et al. 'Potential health benefits of dietary phytoestrogens: a

review of the clinical, epidemiological, and mechanistic evidence'. *Journal of Clinical Endocrinology and Metabolism* 1998; 83(7): 2223–2235.

4. USDA-Iowa State University Database on the Isoflavone Content of Foods – 1999. website address: www.nal.usda.gov/fnic/foodcomp/Data/isoflav/isoflav.html

11 The Value of Isoflavone-rich Supplements

1. Novogen Ltd. 'Clinical evidence that Novogen product protects against bone and heart disease.' Press release 24/9/99.

12 Complementary Therapies and the Menopause

1. Woodham, A. and Peters, D., *Encyclopedia of Complementary Medicine – The Definitive Guide to the Best Treatment Options for 200 Health Problems.* Dorling Kindersley, 1997, pp. 96 & 100.

13 The Benefits of Exercise

1. Notelovitz, M., 'The non-hormonal management of the menopause', in *The Menopause*, Eds. Studd, J.W.W., Whitehead, M.I. Blackwell Scientific Publications, Oxford, 1988.

2. Notelovitz, M., 'The non-hormonal management of the menopause', in *The Modern Management of the Menopause*, edited by G. Berg & M. Hammer, Parthenon Publishing, 1994.

3. Cowan, M.M., Gregory, L.W., 'Responses of pre- and postmenopausal females to aerobic conditioning'. *Medical Science, Sports and Exercise* 1985; 17: 138–43.

4. Morgan, W.P., 'Anxiety reduction following acute physical activity'. *Psychiatry Annals*, 1979; 9: 36–45.

5. Morgan, W.P., et al., 'Facilitation of physical performance by means of cognitive strategy'. *Cognitive Therapy Research* 1983; 7: 251–64.

6. Penny, G.D., Rust, J.O., 'Effect of walking-jogging programme on personality characteristics of middle-aged females'. *Journal of Sports Medicine* 1982; 20: 221–6.

7. Gill, A.A., et al., 'A well woman's health maintenance study comparing physical fitness and group support programs'. *Journal of Occupational Therapy and Research* 1984; 4: 286–308.

8. Greist, J.H., et al., 'Running as treatment for depression'. *Comprehensive Psychiatry* 1979; 20: 41–53.

9. Goldberg, L., et al., 'Changes in lipid and lipoprotein levels after weight training'. *Journal of American Medical Association* 1984; 252: 504–6.

10. Martin, A.D., et al., 'Predicting maximal oxygen uptake from treadmill testing in trained and untrained women'. *American Journal of Obstetrics and Gynaecology* 1989; 161: 127–32.

11. Martin, D., Notelovitz, M., 'Effects of aerobic training on bone mineral density of postmenopausal women'. *Journal of Bone and Mineral Research* 1993; 8: 931–6.

12. Notelovitz, M., et al., 'Cardiorespiratory fitness evaluation in climacteric women: comparison of two methods'. *American Journal of Obstetrics and Gynaecology* 1986; 154: 1009–13.

13. Probart, C.K., et al., 'The effect of moderate aerobic exercise on physical fitness among women 70 years and older'. *Maturitas* 1991; 14: 49–56.

14. Van Dam, S., et al., 'Effect of exercise on glucose metabolism in postmenopausal women'. *American Journal of Obstetrics and Gynaecology* 1988; 159: 82–6.

15. Spiriduso, W.W., 'Exercise as a factor in aging motor behaviour plasticity in exercise and health', in *American Academy of Physical Education Papers 17*, pp. 89–100. Human Kinetics Publishers, Inc., Champaign, Illinois.

16. Spiriduso, W.W., Clifford, P., 'Replication of age and physical activity effects in reaction and movement time'. *Journal of Gerontology* 1978; 33: 26–30.

14 The Benefits of Relaxation

1. Hunter, M.S., 'A treatment option for menopausal hot flushes: cognitive relaxation therapy'. *European Menopause Journal* 1995; 2(3):16–17.

6
CHARTS AND DIARIES

Menopause Symptom Questionnaire

Do you suffer from any of the following? Please ensure each symptom is only ticked *once*.

	* How many times per month	None	Mild	Moderate	Severe
1 Hot/cold flushes*					
2 Facial/body flushing*					
3 Nightsweats*					
4 Palpitations*					
5 Panic attacks*					
6 Generalised aches and pains					
7 Depression					
8 Perspiration					
9 Numbness/skin tingling in arms and legs					
10 Headaches					
11 Backaches					
12 Fatigue					
13 Irritability					
14 Anxiety					
15 Nervousness					
16 Loss of confidence					
17 Insomnia					
18 Giddiness/dizziness					
19 Difficulty/frequency in passing water					
20 Water retention					

21	Bloated abdomen				
22	Constipation				
23	Itchy vagina				
24	Dry vagina				
25	Painful intercourse				
26	Decreased sex drive				
27	Loss of concentration				
28	Confusion/Loss of vitality				

Menopause Symptomatology Daily Diary

Grading of symptoms

0 None
1 Mild – present but does not interfere with activities
2 Moderate – present and interferes with activities but not disabling
3 Severe – disabling. Unable to function

Date																				
Hot/cold flushes*																				
Facial/body flushing*																				
Nightsweats*																				
Palpitations*																				
Panic attacks*																				
Generalised aches and pains																				
Depression																				
Perspiration																				
Numbness/skin tingling in arms and legs																				
Headaches																				
Backaches																				
Fatigue																				
Irritability																				
Anxiety																				
Nervousness																				
Loss of confidence																				

Insomnia	
Giddiness/dizziness	
Difficulty/frequency in passing water	
Constipation	
Itchy vagina	
Dry vagina	
Painful intercourse	
Decreased sex drive	
Loss of concentration	
Weight in pounds	
Notes	

Please complete on a *daily basis* for all food and drink consumed

	BREAKFAST	LUNCH	DINNER	SNACKS
DAY 1				
DAY 2				
DAY 3				

DAY 4	DAY 5	DAY 6	DAY 7

Exercise and Relaxation Chart

Type of exercise and time	Time on Monday	Time on Tuesday	Time on Wednesday	Time on Thursday	Time on Friday	Time on Saturday	Time on Sunday

Type of relaxation							

Once you have completed this for the week, pin it up on a noticeboard or on your fridge and tick off the sessions as you do them.

INDEX OF RECIPES AND INGREDIENTS

Note: see also nutritional plans (main index)

INDEX

Note
page numbers in italics refer to Dictionary of Terms (Appendix 2)